THE ILLUSION OF JUSTICE

An Insider Account of the Greed, Power, and Broken Promises of the NFL Concussion Settlement

CRAIG MITNICK

Rockwater Media books may be purchased in bulk at special discounts for sales promotion, corporate gifts, fund-raising, or educational purposes. Special editions can also be created to specifications. For details, contact the Special Sales Department, Rockwater Media LLC, 109 North Clermont Avenue, Margate City, NJ 08402, 856-427-9000, or craig@craigmitnick.com.

Library of Congress Cataloging-in-Publication Data is available on file.

Cover design by Rockwater Media LLC
Cover illustrations: Getty Images and Shutterstock (gavel)

Hardcopy ISBN: 979-8-9964734-0-3
Paperback ISBN: 979-8-9964734-1-0

EBook ISBN: 979-8-9964734-2-7

Audio Book: ISBN: 979-8-9964734-3-4

Printed in the United States of America

For Kevin Turner and every former NFL player who sacrificed his body and spirit for the game he loved and for the countless families who carried the weight of that sacrifice—their struggles, their silence, and their pain.

To my mother Carol and my father Harvey for their unselfish lives, their unwavering support, and their gift of compassion.

The power of silence can be deafening.
The NFL built an empire. The players paid the price.
The lawyers cashed the check.
The Illusion of Justice is not about touchdowns or trophies.
It is about betrayal, silence, and the human cost of a system built to protect the powerful. It is about men discarded, families shattered, and one attorney's descent into the heart of a scandal that would haunt him forever.
This is a story about power unchecked, about greed masquerading as justice, about lives destroyed not by the hits they took on Sundays, but by the silence that followed.
As the League schemed, as lawyers clawed for position, as players slipped further into dementia, depression, and despair, one lawyer found himself caught between loyalty and survival. He thought he was fighting for what was right. Instead, he discovered just how far ego and money could go to bury the truth.

CONTENTS

This is a work of nonfiction. Certain names and identifying details have been changed to protect individuals' privacy. Every effort has been made to ensure the accuracy of events and legal information described herein. Many of the events described throughout are from the Author's personal recollection of events as he recalls them to be.
Certain scenes are condensed or combined for narrative clarity. Subjective impressions and opinions reflect the Author's perspective.

Portions of the material are based on hundreds of conversations with retired NFL players, their spouses, and their families.

PROLOGUE

INITIALLY, when we met, we appeared to have nothing in common. Kevin was from Alabama, a celebrated University of Alabama football hero. I was from southern New Jersey, recently graduated from law school in DC, and had just moved back home to the Philadelphia area. Kevin was quickly becoming known in the National Football League; I, on the other hand, wasn't even known in the local courthouse. Kevin spoke with a strong southern accent; I spoke with a stronger Philadelphia one. And while Kevin always seemed to have a mouth full of Copenhagen, I only knew Copenhagen as a city.

I have always believed that in life, every death follows its own course, and that when our day arrives, we will hopefully leave this earth peacefully and without unnecessary suffering. I know Kevin shared that same hope. But then, one day, he found his hands less mobile than they had been the day before—one moment believing he was healthy and strong, the next discovering he was suddenly frail and helpless. He had once felt invincible, only to find himself vulnerable—that vulnerability eventually leaving him unable to see or feel the love of his parents or children. When time stood still long enough for Kevin to look at himself in the mirror, he saw someone he didn't recognize, knowing that each day would force him to endure more anguish than the day before, even as he tried to block out the fear of what tomorrow might bring. All in the name of greed, power and money; all in the name of the National Football League. Kevin's debilitating disease, ALS, was anything but random. It was a disease that stole a father from his children and tore a son from his parents. A life and death, like so many others, defined forever by American football.

There are twenty-one thousand retired NFL players living today. Included are those who are not yet sick but wake up every day with the fear of tomorrow; those who have not yet been fully diagnosed but know that day is imminent because of the debilitating migraine headaches they often suffer and their inability to care for themselves in the way they once did. Also included are those suffering from full-blown dementia, Alzheimer's, and Parkinson's disease. Kevin stands as symbolic of all these players, along with the ones who have taken their own lives due to the unbearable pain and hopelessness they felt could not be overcome. Whether Junior Seau or Aaron Hernandez, whether Andre Waters or those less notable players, each of their lives has been altered or stolen forever. They were robbed—all in the name of money and power, greed and ego.

I once said that if there was an award dedicated to the most courageous human beings, Kevin would undoubtedly have been one of the recipients. There is no doubt in my mind that he would then dedicate that award to someone else, possibly some-one he believed to be less fortunate than himself. In my mind, as I revisit my friendship with Kevin, as well as my time with the thousands of other players I was fortunate enough to cross paths with, I cannot fathom anyone being less fortunate than Kevin—or any of the others.

PROLOGUE

. . . and this is what drives me to tell this story and motivates my chase for justice, even knowing that sometimes justice may never be found.

INTRODUCTION

THOUSANDS of young football players who put on a helmet for the first time share the same dream: to one day play in the NFL. The fame and fortune that come with being an NFL player are like no other. The thought of throwing a Super Bowl touchdown or intercepting the ball at a crucial moment are the kinds of dreams kids share across the world. However, the vision of wearing a San Francisco 49ers jersey or getting drafted by the New England Patriots in the first round becomes reality for only a select few.

From backyards to sandlots, from Friday nights under the bleachers to college Saturdays, the dream never dies—it only grows louder. Every boy who tapes his wrists, lines up in the cold, or hears his name echo across a cracked PA system imagines what it would feel like to hear it on a Sunday. The smell of grass, the burn of sweat, the sound of a crowd that believes in you—it becomes a kind of religion long before the paycheck ever arrives.

For those few, the moment their cleats touch the field beneath the glare of Sunday lights, the world stands still. Stadiums roar like living creatures. Every breath, every hit, every yard becomes a story written in sweat. It is the kind of glory that can make a man believe he's immortal. The sound of the crowd, the blinding flash of cameras, the sheer electricity of the game—all of it becomes addictive. On the surface, it is everything a boy could dream of becoming.

But when the lights dim and the last echo of applause fades into the night, another world takes shape—one hidden beneath the roar of the crowd. It's quieter there, lonelier. The sound of tape peeling, the clatter of helmets, the soft grunt of pain that no one hears once the cameras shut off.

Out on the field, the biggest hits draw the biggest cheers. The collisions echo through the stadium like thunder, shaking the ground and rattling the air. Every jarring crack of pads is met with a roar that swells to the heavens—a crowd intoxicated by impact. The harder the fall, the louder the celebration. Pain becomes performance, and the game feeds on those moments—the ones that light up the highlight reels, sell the jerseys, and make legends out of broken bodies. It's beauty and brutality in the same heartbeat. And no matter how many lights flicker behind dazed eyes, the game doesn't stop. It keeps moving—relentless, merciless, unstoppable.

And it is the blood, sweat, and tears of the players—our heroes of the present—that fuel the heartbeat of the game. They are the foundation on which the League's power stands, the living proof of what sacrifice looks like under the brightest lights. Their courage defines Sunday. Their brilliance builds legends. Every yard gained, every hit taken, every roar from the crowd is a tribute to the men who make the impossible look routine.

On any given Sunday, new heroes are born and memories of a lifetime are made. For some players, those memories will be everlasting, preserved in the chronicles of sport. But for others, they will vanish as quickly as they arose.

To the fans, the NFL isn't just a sport—it's a stage for gods. The air crackles with noise, the cameras catch every bead of sweat, and time itself seems to stop when the ball leaves the quarterback's hand. The crowd rises in one voice, a thousand hearts pounding in rhythm with the game. Under the lights, every play feels destined for history. Every hero seems untouchable. And for those few hours on Sunday, the world believes it. They run onto the field like gladiators, each play a test of will, each hit a reminder that the line between triumph and tragedy is paper-thin. The crowd doesn't see the fear or the pain—only the glory.

The noise fades, the lights dim—and somewhere, the dream begins again. In backyards and small-town fields across America, young boys put on their helmets and chase the same dream. The same glory. The cycle begins again—the promise, the cheers, the fall—because some dreams are too bright to see the shadows they cast.

And still, the children dream—chasing the same light, unaware of what waits in the dark beyond it . . .

1

ONE LAST CHANCE

A PLAYER'S HOME IN RURAL AMERICA: SPRING 2009

Life and memories.

THE morning air carried that faint metallic chill before rain. Across the cul-de-sac, sprinklers hummed on autopilot, tossing perfect arcs across perfect lawns. The world outside looked calm, unbothered. No one noticed the blinds stayed closed or that the morning paper was still on the porch.

Inside, the silence had a pulse.

The neighborhood had grown used to it—the quiet, the absence of laughter that once drifted from the backyard where he used to grill with teammates. On Sundays, when TV commentary bled through open windows, his house stayed quiet. The kids who rode bikes past didn't know his name, only that someone famous used to live there.

He'd been the kind of player who filled stadiums—one of those rare bodies built for violence, precision, and grace. Broad-shouldered, fast, fearless. The kind coaches called a "franchise cornerstone." The kind fans believed would live forever.

But forever has an expiration date.

The game had given him everything—glory, money, attention—then quietly taken it back, piece by piece. First came the pain, then the pills, then the fog. Somewhere in the middle, he started to lose himself.

In the quiet of that house, trophies still lined the mantle, gleaming under a thin layer of dust, each one a monument to a life that no longer felt real. Autographed footballs. Championship rings. A jersey folded neatly in a frame, his name stitched bold across the shoulders. They were supposed to mean something.

They were supposed to outlast him.

But what good is legacy when it can't speak back?

Some nights, he'd walk the hallway barefoot, flicking on lights one by one, as if illumination could make the memories behave.

Sometimes he'd talk to himself, half out loud, repeating plays he used to know by heart. The sequence of a blitz. The way a receiver cuts inside on third and short. He still knew those details, still felt the rhythm of the game, even as the rest of his mind betrayed him.

He'd been trained to push through pain. "Shake it off," the coaches used to say. "You're fine." And he always had been—or thought he was. But some injuries you can't stretch out or tape down. The ones behind the eyes don't heal the same way.

In recent months, his reflection had started to feel like a stranger's. The man in the mirror was heavier—not in body, but in spirit. He'd stare at his own eyes and see flashes: a hit he took years ago, the taste of blood, the roar of a crowd fading into static. The past came in fragments now, a film reel out of order.

He'd written notes on sticky pads and taped them to the fridge:

Take medicine. Don't forget to eat. Call her.

Sometimes he'd read them and forget what they meant.

Friends stopped calling—not because they didn't care, but because they didn't know what to say. The man who once carried an entire defense on his back now struggled to remember the day of the week. Pride kept him from answering the phone; shame kept him from asking for help.

But there was one sound that constantly haunted him—the echo of his own name. The announcer's voice booming over a stadium loudspeaker. The crowd chanting, wild with devotion. Those cheers used to make him feel invincible. Now they played on loop in his head, warped and hollow, like ghosts cheering for a man who no longer existed.

It had been weeks since he'd left the house. The calendar on the wall still showed last season. Somewhere in the kitchen, a clock ticked loud enough to drive him mad.

Tick. Tick. Tick.

The sound of time passing him by.

He wandered from room to room, retracing the map of a life he no longer recognized. The living room was still a shrine to his career—photographs, plaques, old game balls. But it all felt foreign now, like someone else's story.

He paused at the stairs, the creak beneath his foot sharp in the silence. His body—once a machine of perfect motion—moved with hesitation. He felt every step in his bones, in the dull ache that crawled up his spine.

And beneath that pain, something darker simmered—the weight of confusion, the exhaustion of pretending, the ache of remembering too much one moment and nothing the next.

He whispered to no one, his voice cracked and thin.

"God, what happened to me?"

But no answer came—only the same stillness that had taken up residence in every corner of that house.

The world outside kept spinning. The league kept playing.

Somewhere, new heroes were rising under the lights. The highlight reels rolled on without him.

And inside that quiet house, another story was beginning—one that no camera would ever capture.

The house sat back from the road, quiet and unremarkable. A gravel driveway crunched beneath the tires of visitors who rarely came. The shutters needed paint, and the lawn bore the patchy neglect of a man who no longer cared about appearances. From the outside, no one would have guessed that inside lived a man who once embodied America's obsession with strength, speed, and glory.

He was thirty-three, though he felt decades older. His knees ached when he climbed the stairs. His head throbbed in unpredictable rhythms—migraines that came on like summer storms: sudden, violent, impossible to stop. And the darkness never let him go.

He wandered through the rooms like a stranger, pausing in front of pictures that had once filled him with pride. A framed newspaper clipping showed him in uniform, leaping to make a tackle. A plaque from his college days carried the words warrior, leader, unstoppable. They had been true once. Now they mocked him.

He touched the frames as if to steady himself. What did it all mean if this was where he had landed—alone in a house that felt more like a cage? The roar of the crowd had vanished, replaced by silence so thick it felt like suffocation.

Downstairs, behind a large-framed photo of himself in mid-play, was the safe. The steel door held memories he wasn't sure he wanted to face. He tugged the photo aside and pressed his fingers against the dial. Numbers slipped from his mind. He tried once, twice, three times. Nothing.

Anger rose, hot and sharp. He stormed upstairs, rifled through his cufflink box, and found the crumpled slip of paper he had tucked away long ago. The numbers were smudged, the ink worn thin but still legible. His hands shook as he descended the stairs again, each step heavier than the last.

The safe clicked open.

Inside were fragments of a life that now felt like fiction: a Super Bowl credential with his name printed in bold, ticket stubs, game programs, photographs. They spilled onto the hardwood floor.

One by one, he picked them up. His draft day photo—his smile stretched wide, his parents beside him, tears in his mother's eyes. Another with three college teammates, arms around each other, full of swagger and youth. And then—his wedding day. His bride's veil blowing in the breeze, her smile radiant, her trust absolute.

He sank onto the floor, photos spread across his lap, and for a fleeting second he tried to summon the feelings those moments once carried. But they were gone. The smiles, the joy, the triumph—vanished like smoke.

He reached inside the safe again and pulled out the handgun. Heavy. Cold. Certain.

He closed his eyes. The prayer rose in his throat before he even realized he was speaking.

"Dear Gracious God, I come to You begging for a moment of stillness in my tears. I am hurting so much that I can't focus on breathing. Come inside my mind and take over. Put Your hands on my shoulders and shake me out of this state. I can't gain control by myself. I need You. Help me gather myself so I can begin to find stability. I need peace in my heart, quietness in my mind. My thoughts are spinning—backward, upside down, I don't know. Please, God, give me grace and help me."

The words hung in the air. No answer. No relief. Just the same crushing silence.

The barrel trembled against his chin. He lowered it to his chest.

One last chance to stop. To put it back. To breathe.

But the hope was gone.

The shot thundered through the house. Birds startled from the trees outside. The gun clattered to the floor, followed by his body.

Upstairs, the baby monitor glowed green, silent. In the driveway, headlights appeared as his wife's car approached. She hummed softly to the infant in the back seat, unaware that inside the house, life as she knew it had already ended.

He was thirty-three—too young to leave the world, too old to believe in fairy tales. His death would be written off as depression, as personal demons, as tragedy without explanation. But it was more than that. It was part of a pattern emerging around the country—an epidemic cloaked in silence.

Other players were suffering too—isolated in their homes, bewildered by memory loss, rage, confusion, depression, and pain. Each believed they were alone. Each carried their burden in silence. Each stared into the abyss with no lifeline to grasp.

The report from the medical examiner would call it a tragedy, but with time the files at the Boston University Brain Lab would call it a pattern.

The funeral was small, chosen by his wife because she couldn't bear the thought of cameras or strangers. Only family, a few teammates, and the closest friends filled the pews in the church overlooking the ocean. The scent of lilies clung to the air, heavy and funereal, mingling with the salt of tears.

His wife sat in the front row, her hands clasped so tightly one would have thought they were going to explode. The baby slept in her mother's arms, unaware of the grief surrounding her—unaware that she would never know her father. Every so often, the wife's lips moved—soft, soundless apologies to the man in the casket.

She held so much guilt, though she had done nothing wrong. She had blamed herself—his distance, his moods, the silence between them. She thought maybe she wasn't good enough anymore. Maybe she had failed him. Now she would never have the chance to ask. She was an NFL player's wife, and she was a saint.

Her face bore the exhaustion of months spent watching him sit in silence—the late-night pacing, the lost words, the forgotten appointments, the blank stares at walls that once held laughter.

Her eyes were a mirror into her soul, and all she could see was what she saw when she came home that tragic night. It would always affect her soul.

When his best friend and teammate stood, the chapel fell still. He had just taken a red-eye flight from across the country to say goodbye. He held the sides of the podium like it was the only thing keeping him upright. For a long time, he said nothing—just stared down at the casket, jaw trembling. When he finally spoke, his voice cracked.

"In life," he began quietly, "you meet a lot of people. Teammates, friends, coworkers. But some of us, if we are fortunate, meet another human being who, with time, becomes part of you. Not just because of shared memories or years spent together, but because they get inside you—into your bones—they change who you are."

He looked down, swallowed, and forced a thin breath through his throat.

"He was that person for me."

A pause. The silence pressed closer.

"We didn't need to talk every day. Some friendships just . . . exist. You pick up the phone after months and it's like no time passed. We had that. But this—" He stopped, shaking his head, eyes wet. "This I never saw coming. And I can't stop thinking—what if he had called me that night? What if he had just said, 'I'm not okay'? Maybe I could have helped. Maybe he'd still be here."

His shoulders trembled as he tried to continue, but the words tangled in his throat.

He rubbed his face with the back of his hand, his voice breaking into a whisper.

"Why did you let the silence win? If only you would have called."

For a moment, his composure faltered completely. He leaned forward, tears spilling freely, words now half-spoken, half-sobbed.

"I'd have done everything—anything—to stop him from feeling that alone."

He tried to say more but couldn't. The sound that escaped him wasn't speech—just a raw, broken exhale. A hand from the first pew—his wife's hand—rose toward him instinctively, trembling.

The friend stepped away from the podium, shoulders shaking, unable to finish.

The silence that followed was heavier than any sermon. He paused, swallowing hard, and then he spoke again.

"He wasn't weak. He was tired. Tired of pretending he was okay. Tired of waking up every morning wondering what piece of himself had gone missing overnight. Some days he couldn't find his keys; other days he couldn't find his peace. The world saw the warrior, the highlight reels, the trophies. But what I saw—what his family saw—was a man trying to understand why the light inside him was dimming when he had done everything right. God, he wanted to live. But he couldn't find his way back."

His words cracked, and the silence afterward was suffocating.

The friend's hand trembled as he looked toward the closed casket.

Afterward, his wife approached the casket. She pressed her palm against the polished wood, tears streaming silently.

"I'm sorry," she whispered again. "I am so sorry."

As the chapel emptied, the widow's voice echoed with the kind of crying that doesn't ask to be comforted—only heard.

Outside, the sky broke open, and rain fell softly across the cemetery grass. Drops tapped against the coffin like a fading heartbeat.

Somewhere beyond the clouds, the League still played on. The cameras still rolled. The crowds still cheered. And the secret that had stolen him remained buried deeper than the man himself.

2

THE OUTSIDER

SOUTH BEACH, MIAMI: WINTER 2012

Trust vs. Power.

THE first thing I notice about Miami in January is the light. It's sharp, theatrical, bouncing off the water like a spotlight reminding northerners why they suffer through blizzards. By the time I landed, the city hummed with energy—vacationers in linen, Wall Street types with expensive sunglasses, and that week, a pack of trial lawyers pretending to be both.

I wasn't there for the sights. I was there because whispers of a class-action lawsuit against the NFL had begun to circle. What started as quiet murmurs—retired players complaining of headaches, memory lapses, darker things—was turning into something bigger. The right lawyers could smell it. The wrong lawyers could taste it.

The Uber from the airport slid along the causeways like a black fin. Downtown rose out of the water—glass towers, a thousand reflections of the same sun. The driver kept Latin music low and kept glancing at me in the mirror, deciding whether to make small talk.

"Business?" he asked finally. "Something like that," I said.

He shrugged, as if everything in this city was business, then pointed toward a row of yachts moored like white teeth. "That's where the real meetings happen."

I had agreed to spend a couple hours after landing with Gene Rockman, a Philadelphia class-action titan, before our scheduled dinner that evening. Prior to traveling to Miami, Gene had invited me to his Fisher Island vacation home, a private enclave with the highest per capita income in America. The kind of place where money didn't just talk—it roared, usually from the deck of a yacht.

The ferry slid away from the mainland, the skyline leaning back as if giving us room. The dockhands didn't shout. They nodded, taking lines, and the only sounds were the hull nudging pilings and the faint hiss of champagne being opened somewhere just out of sight.

Rockman's building had the kind of quiet that costs a fortune. Carpet thick enough to swallow footsteps. Art I recognized from books—pieces that normally live behind glass.

He met me on a balcony overlooking a private sliver of coastline. The sky glowed peach; the water was a mirror. Rockman wore a white shirt unbuttoned at the throat and a watch that flashed like a lighthouse whenever he gestured.

He was already mid-explanation by the time I set my glass down. He spoke with the rhythm of a lecture he'd given a hundred times—the structure of class actions, the moral stakes he assured me he never lost sight of.

"This case," he said, palm open as if displaying it, "is not just big. It's righteous. It can set a standard the league can't ignore."

He was positioning himself as the leader of the anticipated NFL concussion lawsuit. What I didn't realize then was that he was also positioning himself through my personal relationships with former players—lifelong friends.

We ate lunch—fish that tasted like it had swum to the kitchen and asparagus that snapped at the fork. He asked about the players I knew, the families who trusted me. He wanted names—not on paper yet, just in the air between us, as if the syllables themselves could be leveraged.

When he talked about the case, his voice warmed; when he talked about the players, it cooled. Not cruelty. Distance. Like a man describing a mountain he planned to move with blueprints instead of his hands.

He knew I had connections to retired NFL players. After law school, still in my mid-twenties, I worked out at a local gym where several players trained. At first it was small talk between sets, a nod at the bench, a laugh at a bad rep. Over time, those exchanges hardened into friendships—some so strong they became family. Before long, my house had become a team clubhouse, a refuge, the place where walls fell and masks came off.

Sundays after games told the real stories. Win or lose, the doorbell never stopped ringing. Sometimes it felt like half the roster of the Philadelphia Eagles expected to end their night in my living room. Victories shook the walls—music blasting, beers cracking open like punctuation marks, laughter cutting through the night. Wings piled high, Jägermeister shots lined up like soldiers. My house wasn't a house those nights—it was a ritual. A fraternity. A place where friendships grew and memories stacked up like trophies.

There were rituals within the ritual—cold beer, Jäger, wine coolers for the wives, mountains of food. Someone would start a story with "Remember that time . . . ," and we'd groan and cheer because we already knew the ending. I can still see my friends Britt and Bridgette—celebrating an Eagles win and Britt's game ball—smiles so wide you'd think they'd just hit the lottery.

As they celebrated in the back den with a few other linebackers and their wives, the party raged in the other half of the house. Music shook the windows. The night stretched on like it wanted to live forever.

In the years that followed, the friendships only tightened. Many of us traveled with our wives together, toasted the births of our children, took vacations where we caused scenes everyone around us wanted to be part of. We carved memories into stone—or so we believed.

But time has its own playbook. For me, those memories feel like yesterday. For some of my friends, those moments dissolved—not replaced by new ones but swallowed by shadows none of us saw coming.

Minds grew clouded. Words slipped away in conversations.

Patience thinned. But the loyalty never faded.

This was the currency I carried: trust. Real trust. Not contracts or retainers.

They needed that trust. Rockman wanted it. So did the others.

Rockman expected me to bring players to dinner that evening and surround him with celebrities who could bolster his claim to leadership.

After leaving Rockman's home on Fisher Island that afternoon and heading to my hotel on the strip, my phone rang. It was Chris O'Malley's partner, Jon. Everyone knew O'Malley's name. He was class-action royalty—the kind of lawyer who could fill a ballroom just by announcing he might attend.

Jon wasn't inviting me to dinner. He was summoning me.

Dinner with O'Malley in South Beach.

And just like that, dinner with Rockman was out. Dinner with O'Malley was in.

Miami at dusk becomes a different city. The light turns honey-colored; the shadows lengthen enough to disappear inside. The restaurant O'Malley chose was one of those places where the music is too loud and the tables too close—perfect for being seen but barely overheard.

By five, I had checked into my hotel. I had no idea then that several other big-name attorneys were landing in Miami at that very moment. Later I'd learn that these attorneys, who I refer to as the "select few"— had flown in, each intent on planting their flag at the head of the class-action lawsuit.

The lineup read like a roll call of legal celebrities. Rockman—the asbestos pioneer. Tom G—the LA celebrity lawyer immortalized by the film *Erin Brockovich.* Steve Roberts—the Miami powerhouse, master of airline disaster litigation.

Sharks circling the same drop of blood.

They met in private rooms and hotel lobbies, speaking softly but ensuring everyone noticed them. Each believed he was the natural leader. Each despised the others just enough to pretend they were friends. Ego suffocated the air.

And then there was me.

I didn't arrive on a jet. I didn't own a briefcase worth more than a car. What I had was different: real connections to the players. Men with real lives, real families, real suffering. They couldn't fake what I had. And they knew it.

Weeks prior to arriving in Miami, Rockman had invited me to dinner back in Philadelphia. I didn't know him personally yet, just that he was a class-action star with a mixed reputation. We met at a mob-style Italian joint where the garlic knots were as heavy as the clientele. Over veal parmesan, he pitched me his vision for the case. Suing the NFL, he said, would be a windfall—for the lawyers and the players.

I pushed back. "I'm not really interested."

It felt like a money grab, a cynical play by wealthy attorneys eager to get richer while dangling hope in front of desperate retirees.

He insisted that I at least read the packet of medical information he'd brought. That night, I couldn't sleep. I read. And read.

Medical research. Autopsy reports. Early findings. Accounts of players suffering from something far more destructive than bad luck.

I pictured my friends, one by one. Their faces. Their families.

By sunrise, everything had changed. This wasn't about money. It was about truth. And it was about time.

I began speaking with players—old friends, their teammates. Within days, my phone was buzzing nonstop. Quarterbacks. Linemen. Linebackers. Men who had been gods on Sundays now unable to remember their children's names. Men confessing things they'd never told their wives. Men who felt alone in the dark.

They called *me*. Not Rockman. Not Girardi. Not Roberts.

Me.

That didn't sit well with the Select Few.

They believed their names alone would draw the players in. They thought wrong. And each time my phone rang, their resentment thickened.

First came the side glances. Then the whispered comments. Eventually, the hostility surfaced—wrapped in the kind of polite venom only lawyers can master.

They saw me as an intruder. An outsider. A man who hadn't "earned" a seat in their billion-dollar club.

But the truth was simpler: They were jealous.

As the days passed, the tension didn't just build—it thickened like smoke in a room with no exits.

I remember walking into a conference room where the Select Few and their entourages had gathered. The floor was too new. The coffee burnt. Legal pads lined up like props.

The moment I stepped inside, I felt it.

The crackle. The ego. The resentment.

Then it happened. Sol Schwartz, a Philadelphia attorney with confidence to spare, locked eyes with me. Without a word, he grabbed a pencil and hurled it across the room. It hit the table with a crack that echoed like a warning shot.

It wasn't about the pencil. It was a message.

Know your place.

No one told him to calm down. No one laughed it off. They all just watched me, measuring.

I didn't flinch. I picked up the pencil, set it gently at my seat, and said:

"We ready to talk about players, or just about each other?"

A few of them smiled without smiling. Rockman's partner lowered his eyes. Roberts exhaled the way people do when they want to look magnanimous.

The meeting rolled on—motions, venues, PR strategy. The words were about fairness. The music underneath was about control.

An explosion was inevitable. I just didn't know when.

What I couldn't have known was that the explosion wouldn't come from a legal fight over power or money.

It would come from someone much closer. Someone I cared about deeply. That someone was Kevin Turner.

Kevin—the Alabama football hero. Kevin—the fullback who ran through men like he was built from steel. Kevin—who was beginning to lose his battle with ALS.

His story was about to collide with mine and reshape the fate of thousands of retired players.

Kevin and I met years earlier during an offseason when the Eagles picked him up from New England. I expected swagger. I got humility. Within a night, he felt like someone I'd known for years. Easy laughter. Eye contact. No ego. Just Kevin.

We bonded over snowboarding. In the offseason we'd escape to the Pocono Mountains—two guys with boards in the back, music blaring, Kevin belting out songs off-key and fearless. Those rides were never photographed, never recorded. They were ours. Just speed, cold air, and laughter.

Then came the pain. The prescriptions. The pills.

At first, I didn't see the shift.

But one day, Kevin pulled into my driveway with his infant son Nolan in the back seat. His side mirror dangled by a thread. I asked what happened.

"Some lady swerved into me," he said.

But his eyes were distant. Something was wrong.

I still don't know whether someone hit him or he drifted into another lane. It didn't matter. The pills were in the picture—and they were steering more than the wheel.

My wife and I sat up late that night. Addiction isn't weakness; it's pain with nowhere to go. We made a plan. We talked to Kevin's wife, Joyce. Broke the news gently. Asked for understanding.

The real explanation wouldn't come until years later, when the truth about concussions and CTE finally sharpened into focus.

Addiction wasn't the problem. It was a symptom.

Kevin wasn't alone—and that terrified me more than anything.

Back to the present: When I booked my trip to Miami, I intentionally routed myself through Birmingham to visit Kevin.

He picked me up from the airport—just like old times. Except it wasn't like old times.

ALS had begun its quiet assault. Subtle tremors. Muscles not obeying. But Kevin was still Kevin. Teasing me about my luggage. Calling me soft. We drove with the windows down in the cold because tradition mattered to us.

We ate fried catfish and laughed until we cried, then cried until we laughed again. And then we talked about the case—not in legal terms, but in terms of truth.

If the League had known . . . If Kevin had known . . . Would anything have been different?

Silence answered our questions.

After spending the afternoon together, I hugged him goodbye at the airport. Held on a second longer. There was something in his eyes—unfinished, unspoken.

The next time I saw Kevin's name was in a filing. By Steve Roberts. The Miami airline attorney. One of the Select Few. A man who didn't know Kevin—had probably never cared about Kevin—until there was money on the table.

Kevin had been signed. Not by me. Not by someone who knew him or loved him. Signed by someone who learned his name like a stock symbol.

Kevin had already told me he wanted me to represent him but he had to correct something with another lawyer first.

In that moment, when I found out that the lawyer Kevin was referring to was Roberts, I realized the concussion lawsuit wasn't just about brain damage. It was about ego. It was about supremacy. It was about how fast a friend could be taken from you.

It wasn't about right versus wrong. And now it was personal.

Justice wasn't an idea anymore. It was a battlefield. And I was stepping onto it.

After a long day, I walked along Collins Avenue, neon lights unfurling across hotel facades like electric vines. Tourists laughed. The ocean breathed somewhere in the dark. I kept seeing Kevin's face. And that pencil on the conference room table. Every room in Miami had its own gravity that week.

In one room, I sat with a wife whose husband hadn't slept through the night in months. A fresh bruise on her forearm she kept covered even as she reached for water.

She didn't ask for money. She asked whether the man she married was still in there somewhere.

In another room, my friend Rich who flew in to Miami to meet me, a former strong safety who became a coach, gripped the arm of his chair like a steering wheel. "Too many left turns," he said. Then he laughed. Then he didn't.

Pieces of a picture I hadn't wanted to see.

Around them, circling, were the Select Few—driven, egotistical, hungry in ways hunger shouldn't be admired.

The next morning brought another meeting. Same coffee. Same legal pads. Same tightening silence before someone raised a point like a flag. The decision loomed: who would lead, who would follow, and who would be told to stand aside.

I knew my place—at least they thought I should.

I was the man with the phone numbers you couldn't find online.

The man wives trusted when they couldn't find their husbands in their husbands' eyes.

The outsider.

And because the players trusted me, that made me dangerous.

Rockman pulled me aside at one point, hand on my elbow like we were old friends. "We're aligned," he said smoothly. "Let's make sure we stay that way."

"What does aligned mean," I asked, "when there's only one chair at the head of the table?" He smiled the way men smile when they don't intend to answer. "That we can do a lot of good. Provided we don't . . . complicate things." Complications, in his dictionary, meant players with questions. Wives with concerns. Lawyers who didn't salute quickly enough. "I won't be the complication," I said. "I'll be the reason this isn't a disaster." He squeezed my elbow and drifted away.

That afternoon, three calls came from three unfamiliar numbers. Men testing my voice. "I heard you're the one to talk to." "My buddy said you're straight up." "My wife said to call because she doesn't think I'm listening to her anymore."

I took notes until my hand cramped. Promised nothing. Promised everything.

They laughed. They cried. They thanked me in that quiet way men thank you when they're not used to needing help.

If there was a moment I could have walked away, it was then. But I wasn't built that way.

The last dinner in Miami was in a room with glass on three sides and a view of the water so beautiful it bordered on cruel. Partners from Rockman's firm talked discovery plans, but the subtext wasn't discovery—it was money. Control. Power.

"We need a face for this case," someone said. The face has a name: Kevin.

I didn't say that. I said, "We need a heart."

They pretended not to hear.

In my hotel room, I wrote Kevin's name on hotel stationery and stared until it blurred. Then I wrote the names of other men—men who had bled in my kitchen when someone knocked over a glass, men who built cribs with me on Monday mornings because Sunday nights got away from us. I wrote their wives' names. Their children's names.

I couldn't list every man who would call.

But I could list the ones I had promised myself I wouldn't fail.

The ride to the airport was early. The city looked innocent at that hour. Half the people hadn't woken up yet; the other half hadn't gone to bed.

"Good trip?" the driver asked. "Productive," I said. He laughed. "That's not the same thing."

He dropped me at departures.

I stood on the curb with my bag, listening to rolling suitcases, clicking heels, couples arguing softly. Thought of Fisher Island. The pencil on the table. Kevin's hug that lasted a second too long.

The sun rose over the water and made everything glow. Made everything look cleaner than it really was.

They had their jets, their watches, their rooms with the views.

I had a boarding pass and a message box full of men whose lives were unraveling in their hands like old rope.

They could keep calling me the outsider. I would keep showing up anyway. Because whatever this case was about in Miami—the jockeying, the angles, the power—out there, in living rooms and kitchens and bedrooms where the light wasn't theatrical but simply morning, it was about a different kind of ledger. About what we owed each other. About what the game owed the men who built it. About what truth owed to silence.

The week ended. The real fight hadn't even started.

And I was done waiting for a seat at their table. I was bringing my own.

The welcome was polite; the message wasn't: *Know your place.* If the door wouldn't open in Miami, then maybe Philadelphia would give me a key.

3

FROM MIAMI TO THE CITY OF BROTHERLY LOVE

MIAMI AND PHILADELPHIA: SPRING 2012

Betrayal in plain sight.

MIAMI at night feels like a movie set—music spilling from neon-lit bars, luxury cars inching down Ocean Drive like exotic animals on parade. That evening, I was dressed for a dinner meeting I thought might shape the future: my long-anticipated dinner with Chris O'Malley.

Before O'Malley's office reached out, my night had already been spoken for. I had plans with attorney Gene Rockman, who'd secured a reservation at one of Fisher Island's private restaurants. For most people, Fisher Island is a name, not a location—somewhere they'll never step foot.

Accessible only by ferry or private boat, it's the most exclusive ZIP code in America, a sanctuary where hedge fund managers and celebrities dine under chandeliers, insulated from Miami Beach's chaos.

Rockman had chosen the venue with purpose. This wasn't just dinner. It was a declaration. He wanted the conversation to feel elevated, private—wrapped in inevitability. The aim was clear: to gain leverage in his quest to lead the class action. He understood—as did I—that the number of players contacting me had grown beyond what my firm could shoulder alone. An alliance with him, given his résumé, infrastructure, and history in class actions, felt logical and necessary.

Rockman had the experience, the courtroom credibility, the machinery. Sitting down with him to build a partnership seemed inevitable.

Until O'Malley called.

O'Malley's invitation came with different gravity. A nearly one-on-one dinner offered more than partnership. It offered proximity—direct access to the man already maneuvering to become the lead voice in the concussion litigation. It wasn't about collegiality. It was about power.

I canceled on Rockman—decisively, but not lightly. His dinner would have stretched across hours, full of polished stories and carefully weighed words, where progress was measured in centimeters. I had little patience for that.

O'Malley's dinner promised clarity. A chance to look him in the eye and assess the man. To determine whether he was someone I could stand beside—or someone I would eventually need to stand against.

I remember the Uber ride clearly. The skyline glowed behind me, the evening heat still rising from the pavement. I thought about what I was stepping away from—the predictable conversation with Rockman—and what I was stepping toward: a different game entirely, one where O'Malley wasn't another lawyer at the table. He *was* the table.

The breeze off the water smelled of salt and perfume, ambition and ocean. Hostesses glided between tables with practiced half-smiles. Outside, valet parkers moved in a loop—doors, keys, doors, keys—like a dance choreographed for the wealthy.

Inside, low candlelight flickered in glass bowls, illuminating whispered deals, too-loud laughter, promises sealed by a soft clink of glass.

When I arrived, I was greeted by one of O'Malley's law partners from their Wall Street office. We exchanged pleasantries, ordered drinks, and waited.

An hour passed. No O'Malley.

Time moves differently in rooms like that. Minutes don't tick; they smirk. The waiter refilled our water as if refilling the evening itself. My phone buzzed—two players asking if we were still good to talk tomorrow, a wife telling me her husband wasn't sleeping and was scaring her. I answered each one, pretending the empty chair across from me wasn't telling me a story I already knew.

After an hour and a half, O'Malley finally appeared.

He wore a tight black designer shirt, his hair slicked back above a faded goatee. He walked in like he owned the restaurant. And he wasn't alone. On his arm was a woman who could have stopped traffic—long black hair, piercing blue eyes, a velvet top clinging to her like it had been designed around her body. Her presence shifted the entire room without a word.

He didn't apologize. He didn't even slow down.

Heads turned the way they do when someone arrives lit by their own spotlight. The maître d' straightened. The valet outside likely felt it through the glass.

O'Malley introduced himself with a smirk. And then he detonated the evening.

"Change of plans," he said. Instead of dining with me, he and his companion had decided to head to a steakhouse across the street.

"If time permits," he added with a shrug, "maybe we'll circle back for dessert and talk then."

Just like that, he was gone—out the door with the woman on his arm—leaving me with an untouched glass of water and his partner Jon, who looked like he wanted to sink through the floor.

I leaned in. "What the fuck was that?"

Jon exhaled. "That's just Chris."

"Who is she?"

"It's . . . complicated."

"Make it simple."

And he did.

O'Malley's wife and children lived on the New York side of the George Washington Bridge. The woman on his arm—lived on the New Jersey side. Two households. Two lives. One man balancing them like a circus act.

I sat back, incredulous. "If he's willing to fuck his wife over like that, what do you think he's going to do to me?"

Jon didn't answer. He didn't need to.

"I'm no longer interested in doing business with him," I said.

The waiter drifted by, not asking if we were ready to order. He'd seen it before—deals curdling into nothing. Outside, a Lamborghini growled to life. I tossed my napkin on the table and walked into the Miami night. Music from the club next door hit the sidewalk in waves. I kept walking until the sound felt like someone else's heartbeat.

After that night, I had no intention of dealing with O'Malley again. But life takes strange turns. I was already invested in the case—blinded by justice for the players, and yes, the possibility that the case could also put money in my pocket.

There is a specific gravity to a cause. If it's big enough, it bends everything toward it—logic, patience, even contempt. And this cause was massive. Each phone call tightened its pull. Each wife's fear, each confession from a player—each tear I heard but couldn't wipe away—drew me further in.

I knew exactly how often my phone was ringing—constantly.

Player after player reached out. Some with questions. Others with resolve: "I want in." Guys who were scared. Guys who were angry. Guys who knew something was wrong but didn't have words for it yet. I listened to every one.

And I knew something else—the more players who joined, the more pressure mounted on the NFL. Legal pressure. Public pressure. Moral pressure. This wasn't just a lawsuit. It was a movement.

The names filled my yellow pads, then bled into spreadsheets until the cells resembled stadium seating charts. I kept notes the old way—dates, symptoms, family details—because typing felt too clean for something this raw.

"Headaches since '98." "Can't remember garage codes." "Wife sleeps with keys under pillow."

A former lineman whispered, ashamed, that he'd been punching his microwave because he mixed up the shirt buttons again. A quarterback told me he found himself in his driveway at 3 a.m., car running, no idea where he was going or why.

My motivation was already there—rooted in justice, in truth, in doing right by the men who sacrificed everything. But what ignited me, what lit the fuse, was *the Select Few*. Their arrogance. Their games. Their appetite.

Every dismissive glance. Every whispered aside. Every closed-door meeting I wasn't invited to. It all fueled the fire.

So I worked harder. I answered every call, no matter the hour. I didn't just speak to players—I connected with them. Let them know they weren't alone. That someone actually gave a damn.

By the time I left Miami, I had more than four hundred players signed to my name. Four hundred. And that was only the beginning.

I boarded the plane with a mindset I hadn't arrived with. Gone was hesitation, patience, any illusion that this would be a clean fight. I was in it—both feet, no exit strategy. I didn't just believe justice might come. I planned to drag it to the table myself.

On the flight, the cabin lights dimmed. The city receded like a rumor. I scrolled through the list again—names that once flashed across TV screens now staring back at me like a roll call for a different kind of battle. I sent the same text in twenty variations:

I've got you. We're moving. I won't let this stall.

A flight attendant asked if I wanted anything.

"A win," I said.

She smiled, not knowing what I meant.

Three months later, I found myself in the Federal Courthouse on Market Street in Philadelphia. During my last day in Miami, the panel on Multidistrict Litigation had chosen Philadelphia as the venue for the concussion litigation.

The courthouse loomed like a sermon carved in stone. Philadelphia carries its own weather—gray skies with edges. A wind that tugs at your collar like it's reminding you to pay attention. The building stood just blocks from the Liberty Bell and Independence Hall. Inside, the temperature never changes, as if justice prefers climate control.

It was the first formal hearing in what would be named the NFL Retired Players' Concussion Litigation. The atmosphere was electric. Reporters filled the benches. Lawyers whispered strategies. Retired players sat scattered through the room—faces etched with hope, exhaustion, fear.

You could spot the players instantly. They took up space without trying. The lawyers took up space because they'd practiced. A cameraman's lens hunted for storylines; the stories sat in every row. A former safety massaged the bridge of his nose like he could knead the headaches away. Across the aisle, two wives communicated silently with their eyes: You okay? No.

A reporter whispered, "This could change everything." His partner replied, "Or nothing."

Both wrote the same sentence.

I sat with two close friends—Brad, a former linebacker, and Rich, a strong safety. Rich had doubts about the case, and his wife carried even more.

She was afraid it would look like a money grab—that attaching Rich's name to it would stain his legacy. "Players knew they could get hurt," she said. "Why drag this into court?" I told her she was right—players always understood broken bones, torn ligaments, dislocated shoulders. Injuries you could tape, stitch, pop back into place. But concussions were different. Invisible landmines buried in the brain, detonating years later in the cruelest ways—dementia, Alzheimer's, CTE, ALS. Injuries that didn't end careers, but families. Lives.

I explained something else: We believed the NFL had known. Known and concealed it. Told players there was no long-term danger when their own medicals said otherwise. Rich wasn't stepping into this for money. He was stepping in to matter. To leave behind more than tackles and highlight reels. Maybe this case could save one life.

She understood. Just like that. We settled in. Quiet. Waiting.

Gene Rockman sat two rows in front of me, poised like a man waiting for his coronation. He and the other select few Select Few had already agreed on their leadership structure—hours spent negotiating titles and hierarchy. But what they didn't know was that Judge Anita Brody had her own plans.

The courtroom doors opened and shut with a rhythm: click, hush, shuffle. Brad leaned in. "You sure about these guys?" he whispered.

"I think so."

Then the clerk entered. "Any lawyer representing retired players," he announced, "please take a seat in the jury box."

I rose immediately. At the time, I represented over a thousand retired players. This was the moment—to step forward, to stake my claim. Rockman and his cohort assumed they'd lead. The jury box was their stage.

The room rustled with movement. Lawyers filed forward.

I stepped up as well—until Rockman turned, locked eyes with me, and hissed:

"Sit the fuck down."

I froze.

Maybe I misheard. But the look in his eyes told me I hadn't.

"Sit the fuck down," he repeated. "You don't need to move. I've got this covered."

For reasons I still can't fully explain—deference, hesitation, maybe stupidity—I obeyed.

And when I sat, the doors of power closed.

By sitting, I excluded myself from the leadership table. Despite representing more players than any other attorney in that room, I ceded my position to a man already scheming his way to the front.

The sharks smelled blood. And I had opened the wound myself.

The room's sound changed. The judge's bench seemed higher. My throat tasted metallic. Brad and Rich leaned in. "You okay?"

"Fine," I lied.

The Select Few filed into the box like they were boarding a private jet. The box itself looked like a staged photograph, waiting for a caption: *The future of the case.*

The realization hit hard: I was in a shark tank. The lawyers were the sharks. The courtroom was the water. And the currents weren't driven by justice, but by greed and ego.

A reporter glanced at me, typed something, glanced again. I wondered what sentence my obedience had written for me:

Capable. Connected. Not dangerous.

A sentence that lingers long after you speak louder.

The judge entered. Her voice was small, almost delicate, yet somehow larger than everyone in the room. She asked about consolidation, scheduling, leadership. Every answer had two layers: one for the record and one for the room. Rockman held the microphone like it had been built for his hand. Tom G's tie was too bright. Sol Schwartz nodded in rhythms that suggested agreement with himself.

That one moment—me sinking into my seat—would ultimately cost me millions. And worse, it cost me something beyond value: the chance to protect the players who trusted me.

What I didn't know was that I had already been bitten. The wound was open. And there was no going back.

After the hearing, the hallway outside the courtroom became a river. Lawyers drifted in clumps, eddying around cameras and microphones. I shook hands colder than the room should have allowed. A TV reporter asked me for comment. I responded, "Ask the men in there how many players they've spoken to."

And I realized: sound bites and truth rarely shake hands on the first try.

Outside, the Market Street wind cut through my jacket. I called the first player who had ever reached out to me about the case and told him where we stood. He listened. "As long as you're in it," he said, "I'm in it."

I stood beside a trash can with frost along its rim and let that sentence warm me.

That night, back home and miles from the courthouse, I sat with a legal pad and rewound the day. I wrote *sat down* and cir-cled it hard enough to dent the page beneath. Then I wrote what came next—because regret without a plan is self-indulgence:

Call the wives. Call the players. Make the record in public and in private.

I thought about O'Malley's Miami entrance—the girl, the shrug. About Rockman's hiss. About the players watching from the pews as the jury box filled like a stage.

I promised myself that the next time someone told me to sit, I would stand so still they'd have to walk around me.

Philadelphia tells the truth. Brick, grit, history—you can't hide inside it for long.

The next morning, I walked past Independence Hall. Tourists lined up for stories of freedom and signatures. I looked at the old brick and thought about another kind of signature—men signing retainers with hands that shook, their wives steadying the pen.

Freedom doesn't always come with fireworks. Sometimes it's a man choosing not to stay quiet.

Before the hearing the day before, one of the Select Few drifted over with the smile of a man who finds a nickel under a couch he already owns.

"You've got numbers," he said—meaning players. "We've got structure," he added—meaning power. "We should work . . . in harmony."

The word tasted like perfume on concrete.

Had that conversation occurred after the hearing, his words would've been very different.

You see, when the judge entered the courtroom, the Select Few were poised—ready to dictate their leadership terms. Their coronation rehearsed. Their hierarchy drawn.

But the judge had her own script.

"With regards to leadership," she said softly, "as long as Chris O'Malley is the lead attorney, I'm fine with whatever you decide."

Chris O'Malley.

Not one of the Select Few. Not part of their club. A rival.

Silence.

One of his partners rose awkwardly. "Your Honor, Mr. O'Malley had another court appearance and couldn't be here today."

The Select Few looked like children who'd watched their candy snatched away.

The hearing wrapped up neat and tidy—venue chosen, leadership considered, schedules drafted. But the truth was jagged: a room full of men who believed the judge had robbed them. Men certain the role was theirs until it wasn't.

The next day, I boarded a train out of Philadelphia for a deposition in another case. On the train, the city faded into spring light. My reflection shifted as fields gave way to warehouses, bridges, and old towns. My phone buzzed nonstop. I answered every call. Wrote down every name. Built what they couldn't fake—and couldn't buy.

They had the box.

I had the locker room. And the game was far from over.

The handshakes had rules I didn't write. Fine—then I'd build my own field.

4

KINGS HIGHWAY

HADDONFIELD, NEW JERSEY: FALL 2013

We built a ground game.

I'M generally the first one in. The parking lot is still deciding what kind of day it wants to be—frost on the grass in March, heat wiggling off the blacktop in August, rain that can't commit in November. The strip of offices along King's Highway wakes up the same way every morning. The bakery two doors down cracks its door to let out a sweet cloud of cinnamon; the barber drags his A-frame sign onto the sidewalk; and somebody in the accountant's suite drops a box of paperwork that sounds like bones. Inside, the alarm chirps, the motion sensor blinks, and the lights come up one by one.

The office is modest, proud, and warm. Natural colors—beige, black, mahogany—keep the rooms calm even when the phones don't. Diplomas hang straight; family photos lean in from every wall like a second staff that never takes a day off. The furniture is beautiful without being precious: a conference table that forgives coffee rings, chairs that have heard confessions. In the conference room—the war room—two chalkboards run wall-to-wall.

I don't have a huge practice—never pretended to—but it's successful, honest, and mine.

A decent entranceway, glass doors in every office, and a copy room that doubles as a lunchroom where the air smells like printer toner, coffee, and hand sanitizer. The brass letters on the entrance door—MITNICK LAW—aren't fancy, but they do the trick.

It's about 8:15. That buys me forty-five minutes of quiet before the day starts calling itself an emergency.

Eight months into the NFL case, and it's already eating the majority of my life. My phone seems attached to my ear. That's not a complaint; that's inventory. I wake up with the League on my mind and go to sleep replaying names, dates, symptoms. Some nights I dream in checklists. Some nights I dream in helmets.

Before Gene Rockman called me in late 2011, I was mostly in courtrooms on criminal matters—regular people on the wrong end of the system and sometimes the wrong end of their own decisions.

I liked the fight: indictments that needed oxygen, juries that needed a reason to care. I knew judges, court officers, clerks. I knew which assistant prosecutor laughed at my jokes even when she wasn't supposed to. It was a life with a rhythm.

Then the phone rang, and all the old rhythms started sounding wrong.

"Interested in suing the NFL?" Gene asked. I told him I didn't know enough about it, but I'd meet with him. As I described earlier, after agreeing to meet and reviewing the documents he left me with, things changed. I read the papers like a man checking a scratch on his car and realizing it wasn't a scratch. It was the highway underneath.

I read medical files that didn't care how tough a man used to be. I saw scans and lab work and scribbled notes from wives who had learned to write dates in the margins because the brain at their breakfast table had started running without a calendar. I thought about Steve's forgetfulness we used to blame on late nights. Kevin's personality changes we assigned to pain meds. Joe putting a golf club through a windshield and standing there like he didn't know how glass worked. Britt's insomnia and Dennis's change in personality. All the jokes we made to keep breathing. The paperwork Rockman gave me turned the jokes into evidence.

I didn't know class actions. I knew cross-exams. I didn't know how settlement matrices got built or how "common benefit fees" worked. People told me, "Be careful, Craig—those guys are sharks." I said, "I can swim." That was bravado plus ignorance—the worst kind of flotation device.

I open the blinds. King's Highway is doing its thing—delivery truck, coffee line, school-bus brake squeal. The phone's quiet now, but by nine the blinking light will have a personality. I answer a few emails, scan the headlines, sip my coffee that's already too cold, and check the whiteboard that started as a to-do list and turned into a mural.

Shirley's office is next to mine. Closed, lights off. She's punctual unless a doctor's appointment or an emergency with one of her kids intervenes. Across the hall is Tina's room; she files like a magician and swears like a dock worker when the scanner freezes. No light there either. So I walk down the adjacent hallway.

Brad's door is open, either because he was in or he forgot to close it when he left yesterday.

Brad is a wall with a grin. Iowa strong—dark hair, tan complexion, and shoulders so wide the doorframe looks like it gives him permission each time he walks through. He played for the New York Jets and the Philadelphia Eagles, and the weight room never quite left him. He's goofy in the best possible way, the kind of smart that sneaks up on you in the punchline, and loyal to the bone. Women stare at him in a lobby; he never notices.

"Morning, coach," he says from behind a fortress of Post-its. He calls me that sometimes when he's feeling strong. He's a big man in a chair too small for him, pencil behind one ear.

I'd hired Brad several weeks earlier. One afternoon, right before I offered him a job, he'd walked into the office pretending he had a question about a form he received in the mail. He didn't have a question about a form. We went to lunch. He broke down. Marriage on ice. Thoughts confused. Rage he didn't recognize. Depression that had taken over. The night before, he'd opened the safe, taken out a gun, and stood in a room he loved, feeling like the room didn't love him back.

You don't let a friend go home from lunch with that in his pocket.

I offered him a job. I told him I needed help with players because he spoke their language. That was true. It was also true I needed him in a place with light and ringing phones and people who would notice if he didn't show up. He's been with me for three weeks. The Post-its help. We all do what we must to keep the day in the right shape.

By the time we're done bullshitting about the Eagles and whether the coffee from across the street is better than Starbucks, Tina and Shirley walk in together.

Shirley is compact power—red hair, forearms like she's been lifting the office since before I signed the lease, and the presence of a woman who gets three things done while you're still deciding which one to start. She dresses sharp and fitted because, as she likes to say, "Structure calms chaos." She's unflappable, loud with her laugh, and ruthless with a malfunctioning printer. Good looking, brick-house sturdy, and proud of it.

Tina is the counterweight: blonde, composed, and tailored to the inch—cardigan, pencil skirt, heels that click out confidence. She runs player relations, reads a room in a snap, and picks up the phone like it's a scalpel. Conservative at the desk, sure, but outside these walls she swaps the cardigan for leather and a grin that says the night is young. She's disciplined, warm, and aware of the power of presentation. People underestimate her once. Only once.

"Mandatory meeting at ten," I say.

Tina rolls her eyes. "You mean like the other 'mandatory' meetings that lasted two hours and ended with more questions than answers?"

"First of all," Shirley says, dropping her bag, "there were good questions and good answers—especially from me. Second, I'm leaving at one for the doctor, so let's make it tight."

Brad raises his hand. "I'm available all day. As long as lunch is part of the terms and conditions."

"Noted," I say.

In the conference room, we've mounted two monster chalkboards like we're building a war room for a movie about people who can't afford a war room. I printed complaint captions and taped them up in columns. Names. Docket numbers. Ages and time spent playing in the NFL. The chalkboards hold the rest: city after city, player after player. Hall of Famers. Men you never heard of. Famous quarterbacks and special teamers. Guards whose hands are still the size of dictionaries. The board looks like a league photo taken at a distance—a thousand names, some of whom would eventually take their own lives. If I'd known the board was going to show up in *USA Today*, I would have made it look nicer.

The office phone rings more than usual. Word spreads faster than I can keep up with. Some calls are wives who start with "I don't know if this is something" and end an hour later having told me everything. Some are sons who lower their voices without realizing it because a dad who once shook stadiums is now sleeping on the couch. Some are men I watched on Sundays who open with a joke and close with silence.

By ten I'm still staring at the board like it might answer a question it didn't ask. The four of us crowd in with legal pads and coffee. The file cabinets have become a neighborhood: drawers labeled A–D, E–H, I–L, and so on, stuffed with hard files because no matter how many portals they build, I still run on paper.

We sort. Diagnosed here. Undiagnosed there. "Asymptomatic" goes in quotation marks because it's a word that likes to lie. Dementia. Alzheimer's. Parkinson's symptoms. ALS. Headaches that aren't headaches; they're a way of life. Memory that hiccups. Rages that come out of nowhere and leave shame like a puddle you try to step around. We make piles that feel like something between a library and a triage tent.

"Should we make a list of who's press-friendly?" Tina asks, clicking her pen twice per name. "No cameras for the fragile ones. Some people we can invite to tell the truth if they want to."

I nod. "Only volunteers. Nobody gets turned into a headline without saying yes."

We come to a file with a celebrity name—one of those names that could get a president to pick up a phone on the first ring. One of the greatest quarterbacks of all time. He's hesitating. He doesn't want investors reading his name in the same sentence as "cognitive. " His only symptom, he says, is double vision that makes catching a football with his son a negotiation.

"Hold it," I tell Shirley. "We give him some time, but let's do everything we can to get him aboard. Because of his name, it would be good for all the others."

"Also," Brad mutters, "he's someone who could move the needle the second he breathes in the direction of a microphone."

We keep going. I hear my own voice from Miami in my head—those first meetings where I was learning what to ask: Do your arms tingle? Do you walk into a room and forget why? Have you ever been lost on a route you could drive blindfolded? Migraines—how often? Rage—new? Depression—yes or no?

That last one always landed like a bad snap. No one wanted to say yes. But when I said, "A lot of the guys I'm talking to are saying they are," the tone changed. Men told me truths they hadn't told their wives.

Brad taps a folder. "This one needs a call back. He's not sure if staying in the case is going to make him look greedy."

I tell him, "He's not alone, and once the facts come out—absolutely not."

Shirley points at the whiteboard. "Do we keep an 'Unknown' column?"

"We keep it," I say. "And we give it a better name. Call it 'asymptomatic.' These are the men who think they're fine. Alright," I add, "now separate the Pro Bowlers and Hall of Famers."

Tina has a label maker and a sense of mission. The files get neat spines. The drawers start to look like order. The coffee goes cold and turns into iced coffee with no ice.

At noon, we order lunch. Brad tells a story about a special-teams meeting that ends with a coach throwing a chair and everyone moving their feet at the exact same time, like a chorus line. Shirley and Tina counter with a story about a municipal judge whose toupee once slid halfway south during a ruling, and no one moved because nobody knew the rule for toupee emergencies. We laugh because laughter is WD-40 for the human soul.

Shirley leaves for her doctor's appointment, and I spend the rest of the day with Brad and Tina organizing files.

Around 3 p.m., the office falls into that soft buzz where pens move and the phones have learned our names. Tina's line lights up. She gives me a look—one eyebrow, the *this is the one* look—and answers.

"Mitnick Law, this is Tina." A pause. "Doctor, hi. One moment." She hits speaker and slides the handset between us.

The voice is steady, clinical without being cold. Reputable neurologist. Penn Medicine. "I don't want to speak in riddles," he says. "You're collecting a lot of diagnoses—dementia, Alzheimer's, even ALS. Those labels are real, but they're not the root. You need to focus on chronic traumatic encephalopathy. CTE."

He lets the three letters sit there like a gavel.

"Most people haven't heard of it," he continues. "But it's the underlying process we're starting to see in too many former players. Think of those other diagnoses as the faces. CTE is the skull underneath. Repeated head impacts—concussions and the so-called 'sub-concussive' hits—start a degenerative cascade in specific parts of the brain. Over time, it rewires behavior, mood, memory. Sometimes motor function. It's not one bad day. It's erosion."

Brad leans in, jaw tight. Tina takes notes in her neat, relentless hand.

I say what I feel. "I'm not a doctor. I understand words like 'case' and 'burden.' 'Cascade' is new."

He doesn't laugh. "No problem. Here's the other hard part: At this point, we can only prove CTE after death. That makes the living easy to dismiss and the dead easy to ignore." He inhales. "But you asked me what to watch for. Personality change. Impulse control. Rage that doesn't fit the man. Memory slips that look like laziness until they don't. Depression that arrives like a fog and won't leave. If you chase only the labels the insurance companies recognize, you'll miss the story. The story is the hits."

The room goes very still.

"Craig," he says finally, "build your cases around CTE, and let the other diagnoses hang from it like branches. It will help a judge understand the tree."

We thank him. He gives us three articles, two names, and one warning: "The science will move slow. The men won't."

Then the line clicks. Quiet after a truth.

I stare at the chalkboards like they might rearrange themselves. Dementia. ALS. Depression. All of them could be right—and all of them could be wrong.

By 6:15, I lock the door and head up King's Highway. The day has that late-light color that forgives mistakes. Two doors from the office, the park is filling with kids playing football. I pull over for just a moment. Shoulder pads, jerseys tugged over helmets, the smell of cut grass and rubber pellets. A coach crouches to fix a chin strap. A mom unzips a duffel with the efficiency of a field medic. The ball hits a pair of small hands, and those hands lift it like a trophy. The sound of it—all of it—is joy.

And I find myself counting the invisible things.

The taps of helmet on helmet in line drills. The little knocks that don't draw cheers or whistles. The claps on the crown from a proud coach. The collisions that aren't collisions, just repetitions. Raindrops that become a flood.

Would those parents still be here if they knew the bill might arrive in twenty years, stamped past due? Would I have been, at that age, if someone had told me the game could take a name off your tongue and a memory off your wall?

My first instinct is to argue with myself—to say these are kids, these are different rules, this isn't the NFL. Then the neurologist's voice walks back into my head: *It's not one bad day. It's erosion.*

The thought won't leave. Maybe this isn't an NFL story that trickled down. Maybe it's a youth-sports story that grew up and ended up on TV. Soccer headers. Hockey checks. Friday night kickoffs that taste like a rite of passage. Helmets in pee-wee leagues that look just like the ones on Sundays and teach the same lessons: contact is courage, pain is temporary, your team needs you to get up.

America loves that sermon. We've built entire towns on it.

I pull away, and by the time I hit the light at the circle, the case has changed shape. It isn't just a lawsuit; it's a map. If CTE is the trunk, then the branches run everywhere—schools, rinks, practice fields, living rooms where a father stares too long at a fork, kitchen sinks where a mother learns to hide her fear behind a dish towel, VA hospitals where another kind of impact does its own quiet work. Our board in the conference room is one city on a continent I haven't fully seen.

Traffic slows. I think about the father who just lobbed a ball toward his son, and the kid catches it clean, eyes shining. The father lifts both arms like a referee. That sight crushes me and lifts me at the same time. That's the truth of it: The game gives and the game takes; we've just been bad at keeping the books.

The light changes. Cars behind me tap their horns. I pull through the intersection with the day's thoughts still replaying in my head—the kind of thought that turns the next day into a hinge.

The park falls away in the rearview.

The chalkboards are waiting back on King's Highway . . . and so is the flood.

My office became a lifeline . . . but could it stand up to a billion-dollar system of denial?

5

RAINDROPS

THIRTY MILES OUTSIDE SAN DIEGO: SUMMER 2012

One funeral stood in for a thousand.

FUNERALS are supposed to be occasional. One every few years. You wear a suit, tell a story that makes people smile through tears, go home and sleep. In 2012, former NFL players' funerals started showing up more often. Another service. Another program with a photo of a man who looked far too young. Another family staring at dates that don't add up.

This one is thirty miles east of San Diego. Low hills. Wet grass. A cemetery that faces the ocean like it wants answers from it. The rain isn't dramatic. It's steady. The kind that gets under your collar and stays.

Cars file in—black sedans, rental SUVs with barcode stickers, a few dented pickups that look like real life. People step out in dark clothes and the kind of silence that follows a hard hit. Nobody rushes. Nobody checks a phone unless it buzzes.

He wasn't the biggest star. He was the kind of player who did the heavy lifting and let other people spike the ball. He opened holes. He closed gaps. He took impact like a man clocking in. At the grocery store people would say, "I know you," and he would say yes, and lift their kids up like it was nothing. Now there's a temporary sign in the grass with his name and years that don't make sense. Too short. Way too short.

Under a white canopy the coffin waits. Dark wood. Lilies that don't belong in weather like this. Former teammates drift in, built like monuments with soft faces. Wives with their husbands. Kids who aren't sure how to act. The minister checks his notes, not because he doesn't know what to say, but because there's no way to say it right.

A groundskeeper steers his cart along the edge of the road and lifts two fingers from the wheel as the line passes. It's the smallest salute, the kind you give when you don't have the rank for anything bigger.

The first shovel of earth hits the lid, and the sound is a punch in the ribs. "Ashes to ashes, dust to dust." Everyone flinches. Even the guys who don't flinch at anything.

"Would anyone like to share?" the minister asks.

An old coach steps forward. High school. Whistle-and-hat type. No folder. No poem. Just his hand on the wood.

"He was fourteen," the coach says. "He took the hits and helped the kid who missed a block. Years later, when I saw him after a pro game, he still called me Coach. I told him, 'Just show up for the boys.' He did without hesitation, and they stood taller."

The coach steps back. That's enough.

A teammate, late twenties, steps up next. Eyes red and dry from being open too long. He doesn't bother with thc umbrclla.

"You told me the rules," he says, looking at the box. "Play hard. Love your friends. Call your mom back. Respect your dad. When I thought I was done, you said, 'You've got one more play.' We didn't know then that there were hits that kept going after the whistle. We didn't know the game came home and sat on your chest at night."

He puts his palm flat on the lid. One breath. Two. Then tears start rolling from his eyes like a river flowing hard. The entire crowd just stares. For me, there is something different about it when a grown man cries—just something different.

A third man doesn't talk at all. He sets his helmet on the coffin—scarred. Decals scabbed up. Chin strap frayed. His hand stays on the crown for about a minute as if to say: You don't put your helmet down unless you're done.

Rain ticks. Canvas sags. People shift and pretend they're not wiping their faces.

The minister keeps it short. He should. The day doesn't want speeches. Bagpipes come from a phone and crackle into a thin, broken note that fits the weather. The widow stands with her high-school-aged kids pressed against her sides like she's the only thing keeping them vertical.

Before the lowering, the widow's phone buzzes. She hands it to a friend. He listens, glances away for privacy, turns back.

"It's the coroner," he says. "They're asking for permission to send his brain to Boston University for study."

The widow closes her eyes. Someone says, "You don't have to decide right now." She nods. The rain decides to come harder for a minute and then backs off like it remembered its manners.

Across the country, a different weather system is moving. Glass offices. Airport hotels. Law firms buying radio spots and late-night TV. "If you or a loved one played for the NFL . . . " "Sign here." "No fee unless we recover." A lot of noise. Some of it useful. Most of it just noise.

I'm a solo lawyer from New Jersey with a notebook full of names that won't fit in a calendar. Everybody keeps asking the same question in different tones: Is this a money grab, or is this about truth? People who don't know a single player think it's the first. Wives doing dishes at midnight know it's the second. My job is to make the country know it too.

The only way to change the narrative? Pile stories so high they can't be ignored. Get men and their families in rooms. Put microphones in front of them. Don't let the story get polished. Keep it raw. The public can argue with a headline. They cannot argue with a wife who lives with it.

Back at the graveside, the minister brings everyone in. "We commend him," he says. That's it. No decoration. He asks for strength for the family. Mercy for those still fighting. Rest. The word lands heavy and right.

The grounds crew takes over. They're good at this—quiet, respectful, efficient. The straps tighten, the box goes down, the sound of weight meeting clay is a dull drum. No one looks away.

Even the tough ones stare straight through the rain. The widow lifts her hand to the spot where his forehead would be. Then she turns. The kids turn with her.

Hugs. Promises. "Call me." "Text me when you can't sleep." Men linger in the rain like maybe the cold can wake up the part of them that still believes this isn't real. Then they leave too.

People ask later why this funeral hit harder than the others. It isn't just the loss. It's accumulation. The sense that the game turned tax collector. That we're paying a bill nobody saw when they signed. That disease steals years first and then breath. It's sad that a league making billions still hasn't learned how to say, "We're sorry."

The service isn't an argument. It's evidence. If you want to understand the crisis, stand under that canopy for ten minutes. The proof is the widow's face when the call comes from the coroner. The proof is the helmet laid down like a tool that can't help anymore. The proof is the way men built for collision look away from the ground because they don't want to see it close over someone they loved.

Across the country, in New York, O'Malley holds a meeting with the others to discuss strategy. I'm not invited to the table. I'm running on coffee and willpower. No ads. No billboards. No team behind me. Just names, dates, stories, and a belief that the court of public opinion can move a federal court if you give it enough honest material.

I continue meeting with clients, some over the phone and others in person. Players' wives are always with them. Sometimes the man speaks first. Sometimes he can't. Sometimes his wife does, voice low and flat like a nurse giving doses. We list dates. We write down meds. We collect doctor names and medicals. We don't sensationalize. We tell it straight because the straight is shocking.

The more men who sign, the more the story becomes undeniable. The public can dismiss statistics. They can't dismiss a neighbor who moved the forks because her husband kept putting them in the freezer and then forgot why. They can't dismiss a teammate who says, "We didn't know the fight." That sentence travels. Coaches hear it. Owners hear it. Congress hears it. Courts do, too.

Back in New Jersey, I sit in my office with a chalkboard covered in players' names, divided into each specific lawsuit. I meet with Shirley and Tina to separate files of players already sick from others who haven't yet exhibited symptoms.

In the cases of sick players, we review the notes—when the headaches turned from "annoying" to "constant," when memories began to fade, when hands began shaking. We put together facts and draft press releases to place more pressure on the League through the public domain.

Every time someone says, "money grab," I picture the helmet on the coffin and let the image answer. Every time someone says, "safer now," I think about the widow's hand shaking when the coroner asks for the brain. Every time someone says, "the settlement will fix it," I hear the sound of wet earth on wood and remember that checks don't cure amnesia, and lawsuits don't tuck kids in.

Back in San Diego, there's another layer to this day that nobody wants to talk about, but everybody feels. The fear that this is practice for their own future. That the rain, the canopy, the lilies, the straps—one day they'll belong to you.

He stands three rows back on the left. Former safety. Thirty-four. Shoulders still broad, cheeks a little hollower than last season. Hands jammed into pockets like he's trying to keep them from shaking. He's just begun to get severe headaches. He came to the funeral with two teammates and a cousin. He told himself he'd be fine. He's been to funerals before. This one is different. This one feels like a mirror somebody angled at his face.

He misses the reading. He misses the prayer. He misses almost everything the minister says because his mind leaves the canopy and goes to a place that isn't real but feels more real than the grass under his shoes.

It starts with the rain. It doesn't sound like rain anymore. It sounds like applause, far away. Stadium applause that's been dragged through a tunnel and comes out thin and wrong. He looks up and the canopy is gone. The sky is perfect blue—the kind of blue they paint on posters. The air tastes like Gatorade and blood. He is on a field. No one is warming up. The benches are empty. The scoreboard is blank. In the end zone there's a box. Dark wood. He knows what it is, but his mind refuses the words. He walks to it because his legs have always done what he asked even when his head couldn't keep up. Each step rings like cleats on concrete. He puts his hand out to touch the wood and his hand is suddenly small—ten years old, maybe eleven. He pulls back. He knows what a bad sign that is and keeps walking anyway.

He gets close enough to see his name engraved on a plate that flashes and disappears, flashes and disappears, like the sun can't make up its mind. He hears his mother crying, but she isn't in the stands. She's behind him, somewhere he can't turn to. He hears his son—eight years old—ask a question in a whisper: "Do people still clap when the game is over?" And then the boy says, "I don't want anybody to clap."

His chest gets tight. He has passed every baseline test a team ever gave him. He's faked being fine more times than he can count. He told a teammate several weeks earlier, "It's just a headache," and now he can't say it out loud without tasting metal. He forgets the gate code sometimes. He hides it by saying he changed phones. He loses a word and calls it "stress." He tells his wife he's tired and really means he's scared. The field tilts. The box becomes the canopy again. The rain is back. The bagpipes are a phone with bad reception. He can't breathe right. The sound of earth on wood hits him like a blindside he didn't see coming. He grabs the elbow of the man next to him without looking, just for balance. The man doesn't pull away. In his vision, his own helmet sits on his own coffin. The logo is wrong—two teams stitched together like a bad dream. The chin strap is cut. The visor is cracked. His nephew—he doesn't have a nephew, not yet—lays a folded note next to the helmet. The nephew's hand shakes. The note bleeds ink because it's raining there too. He tries to talk himself back. Count something. Breathe in four, out six. The minister's voice filters through like sound coming from underwater: " . . . rest . . . mercy . . . still waters . . . " The words catch on his ribs.

He blinks hard and he's back under the canopy, three rows from the front, the widow holding two kids to her sides like bookends. He swallows. His throat tastes like pennies. He doesn't remember the coach talking. He doesn't remember the teammate. He has been gone long enough for the service to move on without him.

A single detail punches through: wet earth and wet wool and the clean, hospital smell that rain drags out of lilies. That's what does it. Smell takes you home. Smell takes you back to now. He breathes. He says to himself, I am here, I am here, like he's calling his own name in a huddle.

He doesn't tell anyone about the field-vision. Not today. Later he will google symptoms at 2 a.m. and close the laptop when the screen tells him what he already knows and can't say. He will schedule an appointment and cancel it and schedule it again. He will put a Post-it on the dashboard that says, "BUY MILK," and another that says, "DON'T FORGET . . . " He will show up at a meeting somewhere down the line and sign a retainer with a hand that shakes once and then holds steady.

Right now, he just stands in the rain and lets the straps do their work.

The service ends. Nobody claps. Someone says "Amen" like a sigh. People step forward in twos and threes. The helmet stays on the coffin. The lilies take on water until they look like they might tip.

Across the country, lawyers continue booking flights with firm credit cards. Paralegals are building spreadsheets with tabs named "Leads," "Medical," "Media." Someone is writing a radio script with the words "We can help" in it three times. A television producer is googling "football brain" and calling it research.

In the middle of all that noise, there are women at kitchen tables opening envelopes they don't want to open and putting their heads down for a minute before they pick up the phone to call a number that promises a human on the other end.

I don't have a script. I'm trying to find the line where grief ends and work begins, and I keep finding out there isn't one. I'm trying to turn funerals into fuel without losing the respect the day demands. I'm trying to make the country understand that this isn't about hating the game; it's about loving the people who played it.

Some of the men standing at the graveside are seeing what the safety saw. Not all of them. But enough. A kicker stares too long at the mud on his shoes and imagines his own daughter tracing letters on a box. A left guard keeps his eyes up and refuses to look down because if he does, he will see his name on that temporary sign instead. A cornerback keeps checking the perimeter out of habit, and because his chest feels tight and he's afraid if he closes his eyes the field will tilt again. There is nothing dramatic about it. It looks like guys standing in the rain. It feels like a trapdoor opening under your ribs.

The grounds crew finishes. The canopy sighs. The last umbrella snaps closed with a sound like a breath you didn't know you were holding finally let go.

On the drive out, the widow and children pass the florist van arriving late with arrangements that will be left at a plot that no longer needs them. They pass a man in a Chargers hoodie jogging slow with a dog that wants to go faster. They pass a billboard for a casino with an LED jackpot number blinking higher and higher, like money can outpace gravity. The radio ad break starts—sports talk folding into law firm promises, then back to highlights, then to a segment about safety improvements and new testing protocols.

They turn it off and listen to the tires. The tires are honest.

The next morning in Philadelphia, I set up a microphone that feeds into a speaker with a hum and tell the attending retired players and their wives I'm sorry for the hum; we'll work around it. They laugh. Then they talk. They are better than any speechwriter on earth because they don't waste words. "He gets lost in the house." "He forgets the stove." "He yells and doesn't remember it." "He cries when football's on." "He laughs at the wrong places and then looks at me for help." You can hear the room breathe as one when the sentences line up like that. Not because misery loves company. Because truth does.

The funeral on that hill in San Diego keeps traveling. It shows up in the way men stand when they're trying not to cry. It shows up in the way women lean forward when they're trying not to scream. It shows up when a kid corrects a date on a form because he's the one who remembers the doctor's name. It shows up when a former safety sits in the back near the exit and watches the door like the past might walk in.

People keep asking what I need. I want to say, "a time machine," but I say, "your story, as plain as you can tell it." We stack those stories. We make them tall. We make them strong. We build a wall and a bridge out of them at the same time. We hand it to the press. We hand it to the court. We hand it to anyone who will take it and say, "Look. This is real. This is now."

There will be more services. Some in rain. Some under sun that makes the whole thing feel like a trick. Some with cameras. Some with just family and a grounds crew who know when to stand back. There will be more calls from coroners. There will be more decisions nobody is ready for. There will be more men three rows back who leave the room in their minds and walk onto a field where a box waits in the end zone with a plate that flashes their name and then hides it again.

We will not let them make this look normal. We will not call it routine. We will not let anyone reduce it to percentages and payouts. We will use the only leverage we have—the truth told in voices that can't be faked. We will amplify the quiet parts into microphones. We will say the words nobody wants to hear until the people paid to listen can't pretend they didn't.

Rain fell in San Diego because words couldn't.

6

THE WHITEBOARD

BOSTON UNIVERSITY BRAIN LAB, BOSTON: FALL 2017

Strategy vs. Humanity.

THE hallway to the lab smelled faintly of disinfectant and coffee—a blend of sterility and exhaustion. Fluorescent lights hummed overhead. Outside, Boston baked under an autumn sun, but in here it was always the same season—perpetual winter, where everything important happened on ice.

Long panes of glass divided corridor from lab, and behind them: stainless tables, sterile and waiting. A wall clock ticked with the patience of a surgeon. The elevator doors opened, exhaled, and closed again. Another cart squeaked past with boxes stacked two high—dry ice vapor dragging along the floor like low fog. Most hallways point you somewhere; this one pointed inward, toward the part of yourself that weighs truth against comfort and chooses truth anyway.

Dr. Chris Nowinski, PhD pushed open the office door with his shoulder, juggling a notebook in one hand and a phone in the other. He had the calm, deliberate pace of someone who had taught himself to move carefully after years of moving too fast. Harvard football had carved his jaw; pro wrestling chiseled the rest. The accident in the ring—the kick that ended a career and started a mission—had done the quiet carving, the kind that doesn't show until you stare at yourself in the mirror and realize the man looking back is not the one you used to be.

"Morning," he said to the grad student in the office, papers in hand with names of familiar, deceased NFL players.

"Morning," she replied, juggling her stack of paperwork. She advised Doctor Nowinski that new specimens from pathology had just arrived. Two donors. One military, one football."

Chris set down his coffee and the room shifted the way an audience leans in when the lights dim. He shrugged into his sport jacket and checked the labels. Somewhere, a family had signed a piece of paper. Somewhere, a mother had said yes. Somewhere, the last of someone's secrets had arrived.

"Have them begin with the athlete," Chris said.

In a separate part of the hospital, the lab found its rhythm. Steel lids hissed open; cold rushed out and crawled over their wrists. Clipboards clicked. Someone at the far bench set a timer and its red digits began to count down like a quiet threat. In rooms like this, grief gets converted into process: measurements, labels, the choreography of handling what once handled us.

Dr. Ann McKee and her team moved in practiced rhythm—

scalpel, fixative, microtome. Tissue emerged in ribbons thinner than paper, delicate as moth wings. The sections were set onto glass; the glass moved to stains; the stains went hunting for answers in shades of brown.

"Tau accumulation along the depths of sulci," one of the lab interns narrated softly. "Perivascular foci. Irregular distribution consistent with previous cases."

Dr. McKee leaned over the microscope. She didn't blink. She had learned that if you blink at the wrong second, you can miss the thing you owe to the family—the small betrayal of the brain against its former owner. What she saw was familiar. Too familiar.

If the soul leaves a body at death, the story remains. It lodges in folds and fissures, in the tangled scaffolding of nerve and protein. Chronic Traumatic Encephalopathy—CTE—is a clinical phrase, sterile and orderly. What it means in human terms is disassembly. Memory unpinned. Anger arriving without invitation. Headaches like thunderstorms. A man who once set alarms by instinct now standing in the kitchen at 2 a.m., unsure why he'd come.

The reliable laboratory examinations conducted by Dr. McKee and the compassion exhibited by Dr. Nowinski when informing the families was a far cry from the NFL's own handling of the situation.

Before Dr. Nowinski ever suffered a concussion, which propelled him to further his studies into the correlation between brain injury and concussions, the NFL had its own group "studying" the situation. The Mild Traumatic Brain Injury Committee (MTBI) was led by Dr. Elliot Pellman who, contrary to Doctors McKee and Nowinski, specialized in rheumatology (the study of autoimmune and inflammatory conditions). In his role, Dr. Pellman consistently defended the League, even arguing against the findings of Dr. Bennet Omalu, who was the first to discover and publish a medical study on CTE. Dr. Pellman even went so far as to state that, "We [the MTBI] do not believe that the data support the contention that there is a relationship between concussions and dementia-related illness in our players."

As the Roman philosopher Seneca once said, "Time discovers truth."

Back in the office, Chris thought, as he often did, of the ring light and the kick, the weeks that unraveled like yarn, the doctor who said "concussion" and meant fracture in a life. He thought of the first time a family called and asked, "Can you tell me if I'm crazy, or if the game made my husband someone else?" The microscope was a portal and a mirror; every slide showed him the road he'd taken to this room.

Chris turned from his desk and walked to the whiteboard.

In a brain center that changed bodies but not its habits, the whiteboard did the one job rituals always do—it trapped what would otherwise float away. Names had been layered on it for years in erasable marker that never completely erased: initials, ages, notes, and the terrible shorthand of the trade—RB, 47, advanced; LB, 61, severe; WR, 38, suicide. The corners were smudged with ghosts. A worn blue Expo marker lay in the tray like a wand that only conjured bad news.

After reading the prior day's results from the lab, Chris wrote an ID number beside the latest donor, underlined it, and paused with the cap off, lost between duty and mercy. It never got easier to add a name. It shouldn't.

"Chris?" the intern in his office said. "You okay?"

He nodded and capped the pen. "Yeah. Let's finish reviewing the results."

Doctor McKee entered Chris's office and the two of them worked another hour, Dr. McKee cross-checking stains, comparing atlas prints, while Chris lined up photo documentation for the family report that would go out in careful language later. Somewhere in those paragraphs, the lab would say the one thing families craved and feared most: You were not imagining it.

Dr. McKee dictated notes, slow and precise. "Patchy cortical involvement . . . hippocampal change." Her intern dated the forms; the printer spat labels with the relentless cheer of a metronome. In the corner, the timer reached zero and chirped. They didn't flinch.

Chris's phone vibrated, he almost didn't look. Unknown caller. He swiped. "This is Chris."

A woman's voice, tentative and brittle. "Mr. Nowinski?"

"Yes."

"My son's brain was sent to the lab. He played in the NFL for six years, his name is . . . " A rush of breath on the line. "They told me you're the one."

The office went quieter than it already was. Chris stepped into the hall, pressing the phone to his ear like he could steady her by proximity alone. The corridor felt colder, though he knew it wasn't. He stared at a scuffed patch on the baseboard like it could absorb what she was about to say.

"Yes," he said gently. "I reviewed the examination of your son's brain."

"I need to know," she said. "Please. I need to know if there's a reason. I need to know if my boy was still my boy in there, or if . . . if something took him."

Her breath hitched. Grief will do that—turn syllables to tide. He could hear the shape of a kitchen around her: a chair pulled out too quickly, a faucet left dripping, a radio turned low because silence was worse. Somewhere there was a photograph of a kid in a number he grew into. Somewhere there were trophies that didn't know what else to be.

Chris spoke slowly, letting each sentence find ground before he added another. "Your son had severe CTE. Stage three bordering four. The pathology is extensive. It explains—some of it, not all—the headaches, the impulsivity, the anger that didn't make sense. It explains why he became a stranger to himself."

On the other end: a sob caught mid-breath. "He used to call me after practice and tell me about the plays. He used to say, 'Ma, can you believe I get paid to do this?' And then, later, he stopped calling at all. I thought it was me. I thought I lost him because I did something wrong."

"You didn't," Chris said. "You didn't."

"He was my baby," she whispered, and the word hung there like a bridge that couldn't quite reach the other side.

She cried quietly—the kind of cry that makes you want to put a hand through the phone and touch someone's shoulder. He waited. The hallway clock clicked, measuring mercy in seconds. A tech rolled a cart past at the far end and, seeing him, rolled it back again.

"Thank you," she said at last. "For telling me. For giving me something that isn't a headline."

After they hung up, he leaned his head against the cool plaster wall. The steady hum of the building softened. He closed his eyes and saw not diagnoses but faces—dozens of them—men who had been giants in rooms that now felt too small.

He returned to the office, took a photo of the stained slide and report, labeled it, logged it. Process was a raft, and he climbed aboard.

"Let's secure the lab reports ," he said. "Then we'll brief the family liaison."

They worked in silence, then in small talk—the laboratory dialect of kindness. The student told him her grandmother kept a prayer list and had added "the football doctor." Chris smiled without answering. The whiteboard waited.

On the drive home, Boston unspooled in narrow streets and impatient horns. Heat lay on the asphalt in shivers. He passed the ballpark—pilgrims in caps drifting toward the turnstiles—and the sight struck him like a hymn sung off-key but still beloved. His phone buzzed—a text from his wife: Don't forget your shirts at the cleaners. A mundane kindness, an anchor from an ordinary day.

He pulled into the cleaners' lot and let the engine idle, the A/C clicking defiantly. On the radio a host argued about a trade that would fix everything. He stared through the windshield and thought about the board. He pictured the names. He pictured the space left on the bottom right and wondered who it was meant for, as if fate were a clerk assigning appointments.

At home, he hung the shirts on the back of a chair and told his wife about his day. He told her about the tone of a mother's grief, how it differs from the grief of a wife or a child or a teammate. Mothers grieve the future as much as the past. She made tea, handed him a mug, and didn't try to solve anything.

They brushed their teeth, set phones on chargers, orchestrated the small closing rituals of evening. In the dark, he whispered, "They're still exploiting them, you know. The league. The owners. They're still cashing checks while families are cashing out their futures. And tomorrow I'll have to write another name on that board."

She reached for his hand beneath the sheet. "You're doing the work," she said. "You're naming what they won't."

He stared at the ceiling until the room softened around the edges. Sleep arrived in fragments. In one of them, he stood in the lab with a dry marker that would not write, pressing harder and harder until the tip split.

At 5:12 a.m., his phone vibrated on the nightstand. A text from a number he didn't recognize.

You don't know me, but my husband played eight years in the League. He passed yesterday. He didn't know who he was because his dementia was so advanced. He was angry all the time. He went into rages. My children are hurting. They are devastated at the loss of their father, both in life and in death. I'm sorry for writing so early. Another player's wife gave me your name and told me I should talk to you about having his brain examined. We need to know whether he had CTE. Maybe that will help my children understand. The NFL should be held responsible, and I've been told by our attorney that we can simply put in a claim for dementia. I understand that if he had CTE, we couldn't sue anyway. Is that true? Can you help?

He didn't reply right away. He got up, walked to the kitchen, and watched the sky lift slowly from black to blue. The kettle whistled. He poured water over grounds and felt, as he always did on mornings like this, the terrible arithmetic of the day: There would be another name for the board. There would be, before he slept again, the small, irreversible act of writing.

He typed his response: Yes. I can help. Here's what we do first.

Send.

The whiteboard would be waiting, clean except where it wasn't—a field of past tense. By noon, another set of slides would be stained. By evening, he would decide whether to add a line or pretend, for one more day, that the markers could rest.

He parked at the hospital early and sat with the engine off, listening to the cooling tick of the exhaust. On his lap, the notebook lay open to a page he hadn't meant to leave blank. He wrote three words at the top—Listen. Believe. Translate.—because that was the job: listen to the families, believe what they lived, translate what the tissue confessed.

In the elevator, a nurse balanced a cardboard tray of coffees like a magician. "Long day?" she asked.

"They all are," he said, and immediately wished he'd chosen a softer answer.

She nodded in the universal language of people who show up anyway.

In the office, the student had beaten him in. She'd already arranged the findings. "Donor's wife called," she said. "She asked if we could tell her . . . if he knew it was happening while it was happening."

Chris rubbed his temple. "We can tell her what we know," he said. "And we can tell her she wasn't alone."

In the lab, Dr. McKee began again. Stain, rinse, mount. She adjusted the microscope slowly, the focus knob turning like the face of a clock. The field sharpened to a coastline of light and dark; the brown picked out the damage the way tide outlines wreckage. She e felt the marker in her pocket as if it had weight.

This time Dr. McKee stepped to the board and hovered the cap at the edge of the empty corner. The tray held four pens—blue, black, a green no one used, and a red no one wanted. He always chose blue. She told herself it was because blue looked like sky, and sky looked like mercy.

Across the country in Texas, a woman sat in a luxury suite at a stadium and rolled down her sleeve to cover a bruise before anyone noticed. Her name was Bridgette. Her husband's name was Matt. He had played nine years in the League. He wasn't the same man she married.

She watched the field as if it might offer instructions for life beyond it. The glass in front of her reflected her face superimposed on the game, and for a heartbeat she didn't recognize the woman looking back. Down below, the team huddled; on her phone, a draft text waited unsent: He's getting worse. I'm scared. Who do I call? She erased the last line, typed it again, erased it again, then finally hit send to the number a friend's friend had whispered across a kitchen island like contraband.

In Boston, Chris was observing Dr. McKee's examination. His phone, face down on the bench, pulsed once—an LED heartbeat in the quiet room. He didn't hear it at first; the timer had just chirped, and the rinse had to happen now or not at all. The student reached over and slid the phone toward him without a word. He glanced at the preview—Texas area code—and felt the future inch closer.

The board didn't know their names yet. It would.

He uncapped the blue marker. Somewhere in the building, a door shut with a soft, decisive click, and the sound threaded through the lab like a line break. He drew a small square in the lower right—space reserved, a promise to the living and the dead. The phone vibrated again, longer this time, as if insisting. He picked it up.

"Chris," he answered.

A breath. A voice. "My name is Bridgette," she said. "Are you the one who writes the names?"

7

BACK IN TIME

SOUTHERN NEW JERSEY: FALL 2003

Origins and loyalty.

WALKING out of Veterans Stadium into the sprawl of the South Philly parking lot was a ritual. The crowd spilling out of the concrete bowl, the smell of cheesesteaks mixed with spilled beer, the roar still echoing even as the scoreboard went dark. Back then, on game days in Philadelphia, exhaustion didn't matter. You pushed through it. The energy of the city carried you, especially when the Eagles won.

That Sunday in the fall of 2003 was no different—except it was.

The Eagles had just beaten the Cowboys, and in Philadelphia, beating Dallas was more than a victory. It was personal. It meant the week started better, the beer tasted colder, and the city felt lighter.

For me, it meant only one thing: the after-party was going to be kicking at my house.

I wasn't yet married and was living with two close friends—Scott, a linebacker from Notre Dame, and Andy, a defensive lineman from Ohio—both on the active roster with the Philadelphia Eagles. We weren't just roommates; we were friends. We shared rent, meals, and on Monday mornings, hangovers.

By the time we made it back, the routine had already written itself. The pool table was jammed with players and friends. The fire crackled. Bottles of vodka piled up in the trash can, casualties of the celebration. And at the center of it all was the Jäger machine—an old Jägermeister dispenser that kept shots ice-cold, pumping out trouble one pour at a time. Mixing vodka with Jäger isn't recommended, but try telling that to a room full of twenty-something football players fresh off a division win. Three-quarters into the night, Scott was in the bathroom, hugging the toilet like it was his long-lost love.

"Hey, Scotty," one of the guys shouted through the door. "Don't forget to tell her you love her in the morning!"

Scott's muffled groan turned into laughter from the hallway. That scene repeated itself several times that season.

The house was chaos disguised as a home. By the second or third party, the neighbors stopped calling us "those boys on the block" and started calling us "the circus." The floor was permanently sticky from spilled beer. The front door never really closed because too many linebackers had shouldered it open at once. The kitchen table bowed under the weight of beer pong battles that lasted until dawn. Pizza boxes stacked like a leaning tower on the counter, some with slices so petrified they could have doubled as frisbees.

By Monday mornings, the place looked like a frat house had collided with a junkyard. One shoe here, one sock there. Someone's jersey balled up in the fireplace. Half-drunk beers lined the windowsills like trophies. And no matter what, there was always one guy passed out on the couch, snoring away.

Once, Andy fell asleep holding a chicken wing so long it fused into the cushion overnight. The cops became recurring characters. One officer showed up so often he started joking that we should put him on the guest list.

"Boys," he'd say, stepping into the crowded living room. "You know why I'm here."

"Noise?" I'd ask, feigning innocence.

"Noise," he'd nod. "Turn it down a notch and we'll all pretend I wasn't here."

The night he caught Scott stumbling out of the bathroom, clutching the doorframe for dear life, he just smirked. "Looks like you've got bigger problems than me tonight."

"Turn the music down?!" Scott shouted. "Turn the room down—it's spinning!" The officer shook his head, chuckled, and walked out. He never once wrote a ticket. Maybe he liked the show too much.

The parties were legendary. Beer pong tournaments that stretched into the early hours, house rules nobody could remember in the morning, and losers doing ridiculous dares.

One night, Steve lost six games in a row and ended up running around the block naked with a headlamp duct-taped to his forehead while the rest of us cheered him on. The neighbors were furious, but we laughed so hard our sides hurt.

Other nights, the pool table turned into a wrestling mat. A couple of the guys would square off while the rest of us placed bets. They were mountains colliding—beer bottles rattling on the mantle, pizza boxes sliding off counters. Usually, they ended up sprawled on the carpet, laughing too hard to finish. Nobody ever remembered who won.

Somewhere during one of those nights, someone asked about Kevin Turner. He knew Kevin and I were close, and that Kevin had left Philly a couple years earlier to go back home to Alabama. The mention of his name stopped me. I thought about Kevin and our trips to the mountains, barreling down on snowboards like we were invincible teenagers.

"Bet you two idiots were racing down the slopes, weren't you?" someone said, grinning.

"Racing?" I laughed. "We thought we were training for the Olympics. Only difference was, half the time we didn't even make it halfway down without falling on our asses."

I laughed hard remembering it. But underneath, there was silence, too. If only we'd known what was coming for Kevin—for many of them.

The offseason had its own traditions. Rich, my friend from Hawaii, invited Scott and me to Maui. Scott had gone back home to Detroit after the season ended, but we all met up there. Rich was already tan, already grinning, already taking shots at me before I cleared baggage claim.

"Brah," he said, slapping my stomach, "you sure you didn't eat the whole food cart on the flight over?"

That was the start of the "bloat pig" nickname. Every time I dragged myself out of the water, belly hanging just a little too low, they shouted it across the beach. "Bloat pig!" And then they collapsed in the sand laughing. I hated it. And I loved it. That's what friendship was—merciless teasing wrapped in loyalty.

The days were endless beach runs; the nights, endless bar crawls. More than once, we ended up half naked, drunk, playing "catch the bloat pig if you can." And yes, I had to run like hell.

Rich had a way of making sure that no matter what time we got home, we left for the gym by 10 a.m.

Those workouts hurt.

Scott caught a wave surfing and rode it in like a pro. I caught the same wave, lost my balance, and face-planted so hard I came up with sand in my ears. The guys laughed so hard they nearly fell off their boards. "Bloat pig can't swim!" they shouted.

The nickname stuck for the entire trip.

Then there were the Florida Keys trips with Steve and Joe, two offensive linemen built like freight trains. five-foot-eleven, I felt like a little brother hanging with giants. Steve had played ten years in the NFL. Joe was just as massive, just as long, and just as quick with a joke.

The Keys were chaos. One night in Marathon, after a blur of beers and Jäger shots, Joe slapped the bar. "Next round's on me!" he bellowed. Eight shots later, for reasons lost to history, I was naked outside. Someone yelled, "Get him a bike!" and suddenly I was pedaling a stranger's Schwinn in the nude. I made it maybe two feet before flipping over the handlebars and planting myself flat on the asphalt.

"Don't move!" Steve shouted. He and Joe ran into the bar, grabbed pool chalk, and outlined my body like a crime scene. The whole bar poured out to watch. The laughter was volcanic. I couldn't stop laughing either, even as gravel stuck to my skin.

Later that night, someone dared me to jump into the marina. I did. The water was freezing. Joe cannonballed in after me, drenching the dock. Steve stood on the pier, beer in hand, shaking his head. "You two idiots, there are sharks out there." We jumped out so fast we knocked into each other climbing back.

The next morning, I woke up in the dog's bed covered in cheese doodles. They were everywhere—in my ears, up my nose. Nobody would confess to it.

Another night, Steve ordered nachos "the size of Texas." Steve refused to share food. When the nachos arrived, they were legitimately the size of a hubcap. He downed the entire thing in fifteen minutes, wiped his hands on his shorts, and asked the waitress, "What's for dessert?" The look on her face nearly made me spit out my drink.

We tried deep-sea fishing one day. Steve lived in the Keys in the offseason and was an avid fisherman. "Only bloat pig caught nothing," he pointed out. We laughed so hard we nearly tipped the boat.

Those were the days. The laughter was endless, the hangovers survivable, the friendships unbreakable.

We thought it would last forever. But nothing lasts forever.

Within a few years, the memories I still hold vividly began slipping from the very men who made them with me. For Steve. For Joe. For Scott. For Rich. The sharp edges of the nights blurred—not with time, but with the damage football had left behind. What was once laughter and camaraderie often became silence and confusion.

That is the cruelest part: I can remember it like it was yesterday, but the friends who shared it with me can't.

The truth is those times were our refuge. They were wild, messy, and unforgettable—our way of feeling untouchable for a little while longer. The laughter covered the bruises. The music drowned out the whispers of what the game was already doing to their bodies and minds.

What made those nights extraordinary was how different we all were. They were professional athletes, men who had bled and sacrificed on fields in front of roaring crowds. I wasn't one of them. I didn't wear pads; I didn't hear the crack of helmets every Sunday. My name never appeared on a jersey. But inside those walls, none of that mattered. The distinctions faded under the laughter, under the unspoken bond of being young, reckless, and alive.

Loyalty. Trust. Friendship. That invisible thread tied us together. We needed each other then more than we knew, and even now, I realize it was that bond that made those memories glow brighter than any stadium lights. At the time, we thought we were just living. Looking back, I see it differently. We were trying to outrun something we couldn't see, something waiting in the years ahead.

The cruel irony: Those nights of laughter became the very memories lost for some of the guys. For me, they're frozen in perfect detail. For them, the game erased the reel, leaving only fragments.

The joy that built our loyalty is the reason I won't quit.

Those men taught me more about humility and heart than any courtroom ever could. I learned that people, no matter how strong they appear, carry fragility beneath the surface. Professional athletes aren't just icons; they're human beings. They laugh, they cry, they bleed, and they break like anyone else. When you take the time to see them for who they really are—not the helmets, not the stats, not the highlight reels—you begin to see things differently. That's the truth I carry from those days—the unspoken bond that outlasted the game itself.

Those same friendships drew me into the fight that would follow. They became my reason, my evidence, my cause. When the NFL litigation began, it wasn't about headlines; it was about the men behind those memories. I knew their laughter, their pain, their confusion when their memories began to blur. I had seen what the game gave them, and what it took away. In the end, it wasn't the law that brought me into that fight—it was loyalty. The same loyalty that started in a crowded South Philly living room and has never left me since.

8

IN THE TRENCHES

ACROSS AMERICA: SPRING 2014

The fight itself.

BY the spring of 2014, the lawsuit was no longer just whispers in legal circles or quiet phone calls from desperate wives. It had become national headlines. A cause. A spectacle. America's sport was being dragged into court, and the world wanted to know if its heroes had been sacrificed for profit.

The story lived everywhere—on tickers that crawled beneath late-night highlights, on morning shows where a host's eyebrows tried to signal empathy, on sports radio where callers swung between denial and fury. Airports played it on mute while travelers sipped burnt coffee and glanced up at the subtitles: NFL . . . Concussion . . . Settlement. It felt surreal, watching a fight that had lived in homes throughout the country—inside kitchens and living rooms and hospital corridors—ascend to the jumbotron of American attention.

When word broke that Chris O'Malley had negotiated a preliminary settlement with the NFL, my phone erupted. Reporters, players, wives—everyone wanted clarity. Everyone wanted assurance. And before I could even catch my breath, for the first time since our brief encounter in Miami twenty-four months earlier, O'Malley himself called.

Months earlier, in that Philadelphia federal courtroom at the first hearing, Rockman and the other attorneys strode confidently toward the jury box, certain their leadership roles were all but guaranteed. When the leadership role was handed to Chris O'Malley, the room was turned upside down. As I mentioned earlier, O'Malley wasn't even in the courthouse that day; absence didn't trouble the judge in the slightest. From that moment, the case shifted. O'Malley seized control and almost immediately began private negotiations with the League, cutting the others out entirely. That was when the preliminary settlement was struck—and when my phone rang. It was April 2014.

"Craig," he said, in that smooth, persuasive tone lawyers use when they're about to sell you something, "I need you to help in educating the players and gaining their endorsement as to the terms of the settlement. You're the bridge. You've got their trust."

"You are the only one who can do this," he added, stressing how critically important player buy-in was to the settlement eventually being approved by the court.

What he didn't say—but what I would later understand—was that I was being drafted into a role I never asked for: salesman of someone else's deal, a pawn in a game of billions.

The next two and a half years blurred into airports, hotel conference rooms, and players' homes. I learned the choreography of the road. Middle seats and stale pretzels. The click of retractable banners in ballrooms that smelled like yesterday's coffee. Lanyards that flipped backward and hid your name at the exact moment someone needed to read it.

I stood behind podiums facing rows of men with hands like sledgehammers who now trembled as they held coffee cups. I looked into the faces of retired linebackers in Houston who couldn't remember which child had driven them there. I shook hands with men whose wives stood close, like bodyguards, ready to jump in if confusion turned into anger.

In New York, during Super Bowl week, I stood before a packed room of players. Cameras popped like firecrackers, microphones pushed toward my face, voices buzzed at the edges. But my eyes kept drifting to the back row. Chris O'Malley was there, flanked by two of his associates, watching me quietly. He didn't take notes, didn't interrupt—just sat with that unreadable look, as if weighing every word.

I spoke the way I always did—with preparation and honesty, ready to field whatever came. For an hour and a half, the questions came rapid-fire: medical issues, claims process, timelines, appeals. I answered each one, steady, confident. Then a man I didn't recognize stood up. He was a former player, probably forty-five or so, his body still carrying the frame of Sundays past, but his voice came hard.

"Tell us," the player asked, "how do the lawyers get paid?"

It was the first time anyone had asked me that, and for a split second, the room shifted. Eyes turned sharper, ears leaned closer. I began to explain—the prepaid fund built into the settlement, money the NFL had placed aside to compensate the lawyers who worked for the class as a whole. But before I could finish, he cut me off.

"You're lying," he snapped, voice rising. "All of you lawyers are thieves. This case is going to make you rich while we all continue to deteriorate."

What I didn't know at the time was that he would become the face of the players who objected to the settlement. It just so happened that months later, pictures of the two of us would appear, facing one another like boxers promoting a fight, in a headline article in USA Today.

After he made the "lawyers are thieves" comment, the air went heavy. Players muttered. A few nodded, some glared. My pulse jumped. My face burned. I fought back, my voice climbing over his—louder, sharper—until I was nearly shouting.

"This case is for the players. It's not for us—it's for you, for every man who was left broken by the league."

The words rang out, but even as I said them, I felt the sting.

Looking back, I know he wasn't completely wrong. I thought the enemy was the man standing there challenging me. The truth was harder—the system itself was the enemy, and I was caught inside it.

When the session finally ended, O'Malley made his way forward through the crowd. He shook my hand, his grip firm, his voice calm. "You did well," he said. "Don't let that guy get to you. He doesn't know what he's talking about."

I thanked O'Malley for the support. But long after the room emptied, the player's words stayed with me, echoing louder than the applause, sharper than the cameras' flash.

Months later, in Canton, Ohio, at the Hall of Fame, the irony was unbearable. Busts of legends lined the halls, frozen in bronze glory, while just a few feet away their living counterparts shuffled in wearing name tags because they couldn't trust themselves to remember their own names. Wives whispered to me in hallways: "We've taken his keys away." "He's scaring the kids." "We can't keep living like this."

Everywhere I went, the stories were the same.

Life isn't treating me that well these days.

I lose track of time.

I get lost driving.

Sometimes I don't recognize my own reflection.

And in every city, I carried O'Malley's message: This settlement is the best path forward. Trust me. Trust us.

The players did trust me. That was the part that broke me later.

They called me "brother." They invited me into their homes, shared their family meals, let me into their lives. They told me things they hadn't told their doctors. I was their confessor, their counselor, their last lifeline. I was retained by everyone from famous quarterbacks to other high-profile receivers and linemen, and all I wanted to believe was that I was bringing them salvation.

But looking back, doubts crept in.

They didn't come as thunder; they came like a drip behind a wall. A definition here that didn't match a diagnosis there. A processing timeline that ballooned from weeks to months to a shrug. A clause that read different after midnight. I would stand in front of players and their wives, explaining the settlement, the benefits, the process. Looking back, I now realize that when I spoke, I should have heard the hollow echo of my own words.

One night, in a hotel room outside Chicago, I stared at the settlement documents spread across my bed. The numbers looked neat, clean, definitive. But I could still hear the voice of a wife in San Diego:

"They told me his headaches were just stress. Now he can't tie his own shoes. His teammate and good friend, Junior Seau, recently committed suicide. Where is the help? What is taking so long?"

I poured a drink and asked myself out loud: Am I helping them, or am I delivering them into a trap?

Each time there was a question I was not sure how to answer, I would call O'Malley. He would tell me what to say. I realized later that truth or accuracy apparently was of little importance to him.

There were calls he took on the first ring and calls he didn't return for days at a time. He would tell me things like: "Judge is pleased." "NFL is committed." "You can trust me." Phrases like soft pillows you can sink into and not notice you're falling asleep in the wrong room.

I remember one stop in particular—an NFL alumni chapter meeting in Dayton, Ohio.

The room wasn't flashy: low ceiling, folding chairs lined tight, a coffee urn in the corner that smelled burned by mid-morning. But the men inside gave it weight. Gray hair, stiff gaits, old injuries that never healed right. They carried themselves like they still belonged in shoulder pads, but their eyes told a different story—suspicion, fatigue, a guarded kind of hope.

The questions came at me one after another, voices sharp, not because they didn't care but because they cared too much. They weren't there for speeches or polished lines. They wanted truth. And then one of them stood up, arms folded across his chest.

"Who are the doctors?" he asked. His voice cut through the room. "The ones doing these baseline exams. Are they the league's guys?"

I could feel the ripple go through the group. This wasn't a casual question. Apparently, they'd been talking about it in parking lots, over beers, on late-night phone calls. The fear was alive in the room: that the very exams meant to determine their futures would be run by men already wearing the NFL's colors. That the deck would be stacked before they even sat down in a waiting room.

My mouth went dry. I hadn't been asked that before. And the truth was, I didn't know. Every eye in that room was on me, and for the first time that day, I didn't have an answer. So I took a break and stepped outside.

I called O'Malley. He picked up. His voice came calm, practiced, almost reassuring.

"Don't worry about it," he said. "The doctors are independent. No ties to the NFL. They're coming from major insurance networks—household names, companies everyone knows and trusts. Reputable outfits. The players will be fine."

I clung to those words like a lifeline. I needed them to be true. I walked back into that room, and every head turned to me. You could feel the weight of their stares, like linemen across the line waiting to see your first move.

I repeated Chris's words exactly. "The doctors are independent. No connection to the league. They're coming from national insurance companies, names you know, names you can trust."

For a moment, the tension cracked. Some men nodded. A few leaned back in their chairs. The room exhaled. I believed what I was saying. And because I believed it, they believed me.

But here's what I didn't know—the truth hidden in the fine print of the settlement: Every single doctor, every so-called "independent" examiner, had to be approved by the NFL. Independence was an illusion, written in ink by the very people these men no longer trusted.

So when I stood in that room in Dayton, my voice steady, my words meant to reassure, what I was really doing was something far different. I wasn't giving them truth. I wasn't giving them certainty. I was unknowingly carrying the NFL's message straight into the hearts of men who already feared that the game was rigged against them.

And the worst part? Even though those words weren't mine, they came from my mouth. And once they did, I owned them.

I kept going. I spoke with thousands of players over the time I traveled. In the end, over 99 percent of the twenty-one thousand retired players throughout the country endorsed the settlement.

Ninety-nine percent. A number so high it seemed impossible. And yet it was true.

Everyone took credit for the endorsement rate. One attorney actually clapped. I didn't. I thought of a man in Phoenix who had asked me to write his children's birthdays on an index card so he could practice them. I thought of a wife in Charlotte who pressed a Post-it into my hand that read, please tell him this will not take forever. I carried that note in my wallet until the ink bled into the paper like it was crying.

The 99 percent endorsement guaranteed court approval. It guaranteed O'Malley his payday. And it guaranteed the NFL something far more valuable: protection.

According to O'Malley, my efforts would be nicely rewarded. The settlement contained a clause where $112 million was to be set aside for the attorneys who performed important roles in the lawsuit. Privately, I was told by O'Malley that I would receive a large chunk of money for my role and—more importantly—my results. The money would come from the $112 million paid by the NFL. These funds are known as common benefit monies. I quickly forgot my own words, the ones I uttered in Miami several years earlier: If he would fuck his wife that bad, what's he going to do to me?

I told myself I was being cynical then, that the past didn't have to predict the future. I told myself the cause had burned off the impurities in the men who led it. I told myself a lot of things that sounded like wisdom and functioned like anesthesia.

For me, the realization came slowly, then all at once. I had been the perfect messenger. I had been the bridge, the pawn, the puppet. I had sold the deal, not for the benefit of the players I loved, but for the silent intentions of men who viewed them as numbers, as obstacles, as liabilities. I sold the deal to protect the NFL from other lawsuits—ones with far higher financial rewards. Lawsuits based not on dementia or Alzheimer's, but on a far more serious disease: CTE. When the settlement received final approval, the League could never be held responsible for CTE—a disease that could have wiped them out financially.

I thought I was in the trenches, fighting alongside the players. But the truth was harsher: I had been marching them into a battlefield already lost.

Looking back now, I can still see their faces. The player who couldn't hold a pen steady enough to sign his name. The wife who pressed her palm against her husband's thigh during my speech, as if to anchor him to the present moment. The son who asked me, "Will my dad ever be normal again?"

I answered as best I could. I believed what I was saying.

In the trenches, you don't always realize when you've been flanked. You don't always know until it's too late that the enemy isn't just across the line—it's standing beside you, smiling, shaking your hand with one palm while the other quietly removes your ammunition.

That moment arrived in a beige hotel lobby in Austin, Texas. I had just finished a session—two and a half hours of questions, two hours of hope—when my phone buzzed with an email from O'Malley's office.

Going forward, all communications with class members should be coordinated through... Please refrain from independent outreach that may cause confusion.

I read it twice. I looked up. Across the lobby, a lineman and his wife were waiting for me to help them fill out a medical release. I slipped the phone back into my pocket and walked toward them.

In Phoenix, I explained sympathetically why a specific diagnosis "did not meet criteria." In Denver, a player waved the settlement guidelines like a surrender flag and said, "If I don't fit into one of these boxes, you can't help me, can you?" Men were being sorted like mail. Families were being asked to prove their own pain in fonts and margins determined by people who would never visit their homes.

The nights got heavier. After meetings, players and wives would keep me in doorways with the intimacy of people who want you to stay just a few minutes longer because your leaving means the house goes back to being haunted. "We trust you," they'd say. "Don't let them forget us." I promised I wouldn't. It felt like signing a second retainer—this one with my soul.

One morning, in a Newark conference room, I asked O'Malley for written confirmation of the compensation he'd promised. "Craig," he said, smiling as if I'd told a joke, "Gene Rockman is going to shit when he sees how much money you receive in common benefit monies. What do you need paper for?" He laughed again, the kind of laugh someone uses when they're agreeing to ignore the truth together.

I flew to Minnesota that afternoon and sat at a kitchen table with a player who had caught passes in January games so cold the ball felt like a weapon. He stared at me over the rim of his mug. "If they're going to deny me when I file a claim," he said, "just tell me. Don't make my wife call a stranger to find out what's wrong with me." His wife squeezed his shoulder and looked at me like I had the answer in my pocket next to the email I was pretending not to feel.

The settlement machinery was being prepared for final approval and spun faster. Portals opened; portals crashed. Doctors who had cheered the agreement were now reading footnotes out loud with their palms up, saying, "This dementia definition is not in line with medical standards. It's far more restrictive." The league's statements grew more triumphant as the families grew more tired.

O'Malley's updates kept finding new ways to define "progress."

I was hoping eventually there would be victories—men easily approved, checks that would arrive quickly. I would celebrate those wins with everything I had. But some days, those hopeful wins felt like postcards from a country most couldn't afford to visit.

Back in Philadelphia, the court calendar lurched forward and paused, then forward again. I called O'Malley: Players need timelines. They need certainty. They need to know why approvals are crawling and appeals keep appearing. The reply was a sugar-coated blunt object: Appreciate your passion, Craig. Please direct inquiries through the designated channels. The designated channels were a cul-de-sac.

Then came the call I can't forget. A wife in Ohio, voice raw from sleep and fear. "He's in the garage," she said. "He's just sitting there. He won't come in. He says the game took his name." I kept her on the line until the sun came up, until the neighbors woke, until the garage door creaked and she whispered, "He's coming in now." We never talked about the settlement once. We talked about how to make pancakes without waking the kids, how to put bad thoughts in the laundry with the towels and wash them on hot.

In San Diego, after a meeting that went too long, a former cornerback pulled me aside and held my gaze for a long time. "You're different," he said. "You feel like one of us." Then he added, almost kindly, "That's why they'll turn on you."

I laughed then. I don't laugh at that line anymore.

Winter rolled into spring and then back into winter. The case matured, the appeals to higher courts were getting denied. The press moved on to other scandals. The calls didn't stop. Whenever I pressed too hard, the same language arrived from O'Malley: Thank you for your loyalty, Craig. We've got this now. When I asked to speak at the next hearing, there was no reply. When I pushed for a seat at a leadership meeting, I received a calendar invite with no location. When I followed up, the link had expired.

Somewhere along that road, the trench I thought I was fighting from became a ditch I was being buried in.

The last time I met O'Malley face-to-face during that stretch was in a corner of a midtown restaurant built to make men feel important. He ordered for the table like a benevolent emperor and described the coming months like a weather forecast only he could interpret. When I asked again—politely—for writing on what I was expected to receive, he smiled with his eyes, not his mouth.

"Craig," he said, "don't make this transactional."

I stared at the linen napkin in my lap and thought about all the transactions already completed with the bodies and minds of the men whose wives still texted me at 2 a.m. I paid my own Uber fare home.

By the spring of 2015, the road shows slowed. The machine was built; the lever had been pulled. My lists were now mostly follow-ups, mostly triage. I sat with a father in Tampa who wrote his daughter's name on his palm every morning so he could read it before she walked into the kitchen. I stood in a driveway in San Jose with a man who kept opening and closing the trunk of his car like the answer might be in there if he opened it enough times. I learned how to say, "I'm with you," a dozen ways that didn't sound like a line.

And yet, for all the hours, for all the rooms, for all the hands I held, I could feel the ground shifting beneath me. The promises I had believed—both for the players and for myself—were now shadows passing behind frosted glass. The settlement I had sold like a lifeline was, for too many, becoming a labyrinth.

One afternoon, I opened an envelope sent to me by O'Malley that should have carried momentum but instead contained a new set of rules. They were written in the same polite brutality as always, specifying thresholds and proofs, converting pain into decimals, memory into margins. I put the pages down, stood up, and walked outside. I stood in the yard and listened to the ordinary sounds of my neighborhood—garbage truck, bark, bicycle tire on gravel—and I realized how extraordinary it is when a life is still ordinary.

Because in the trenches, when you finally realize you've been flanked, you have two choices: Keep marching in the direction you were pointed or turn and face what's beside you.

I was about to turn.

And somewhere, on a calendar I hadn't been invited to see, a meeting was scheduled that would decide who got paid for building the bridge—and who got left beneath it.

9

BEHIND CLOSED DOORS

ARLINGTON, TEXAS: FALL 2017

Secrets and deals.

AUTHOR'S NOTE: The following chapter is partially based on compilations from numerous conversations I have had with retired players and their spouses. These stories are examples of real-life scenarios that many NFL players and their families have experienced when dealing with the effects of concussions and CTE. The number one comment that I have heard several hundred times from wives of NFL players is, "I'm not sure who he is, but he's not the man I married."

Sunday in Texas is not a day—it's a ritual. Highways jam with caravans of SUVs flying team flags, tailgates drop to reveal grills already smoking by 10 a.m., and the air carries that strange blend of mesquite and anticipation. Football is church, and the stadium is the cathedral.

In Arlington, the cathedral was a colossus of glass and steel, a monument to spectacle. Inside, the field glittered under stadium lights even though the sun outside was still high. The Dallas Cowboys were hosting, and with them came pageantry—cheerleaders, fireworks, an army of staff moving like clockwork.

For players, though, Sunday wasn't magic. It was obligation.

Matt—a veteran offensive lineman—had spent the night before under curfew at a Holiday Inn, one of the strange indignities of professional football. You could be a millionaire, a father of three, but on Saturday nights before a game, you were treated like a teenager at summer camp. Lights out. Team rules. No exceptions. Of course, these rules only pertained to current players on the roster.

By kickoff, the wives and families had taken their places in the exclusive family suite—a room with leather chairs, flat screens mounted at every angle, and catering that was supposed to make up for the isolation. The women sipped wine, swapped stories about schools and vacations, smiled politely while watching their husbands get battered below.

But in the far corner of the suite, Bridgette wasn't watching the field.

She sat close to Kelly, a defensive back's wife, her eyes hidden behind dark glasses even though they were indoors. When Kelly leaned closer, Bridgette lifted her sleeve. Beneath the fabric was a welt, deep purple and yellow at the edges, raw in the middle. Kelly inhaled sharply.

"Bridgette . . . " she whispered.

Bridgette pulled the sleeve back down. Her voice was low, measured, like someone who had practiced these words but never believed she'd speak them. "He's not the man I married. I don't even recognize him anymore."

Kelly tried to protest—tried to summon a smile, a reassurance—but Bridgette pressed on.

"The anger comes out of nowhere. Rage. He forgets things. He's impulsive. And when he's not in a rage, he's depressed. The kids are scared. I'm scared."

Tears slipped from beneath Bridgette's glasses. She brushed them away quickly, the way wives of players learned to do—silently, invisibly, because appearances mattered almost as much as performance.

Kelly reached for her hand, squeezed it tight. She wanted to say, Leave. Run. Save yourself. But she also knew what Bridgette knew: Love complicates escape, and fear paralyzes even the strongest.

The suite door clicked open and shut, open and shut—ushers, sponsors, security drifting in and out like tides. A PR woman with a laminated credential smiled through the glass; her smile said, *everything here is perfect*, and her eyes said, *if it isn't, don't let me hear it*. Kelly shifted, angling her body to shield Bridgette from view.

The suite erupted as the crowd roared below. A touchdown. Fireworks. Music blaring. The wives stood, clapped, cheered. Bridgette stayed seated, her face expressionless. For her, the game wasn't a celebration anymore. It was a reminder of what football was stealing away.

On the field, Matt crouched in the huddle, his breath ragged through the facemask. His teammates slapped his shoulder pads, shouted calls. He tried to focus, to drown out the static inside his skull.

The crowd noise blurred. His vision narrowed. For a split second, he thought about Bridgette in the suite, about the look she'd given him that morning when he left the house. He didn't know how to make it right.

But he did know why he wasn't right anymore. He was aware of the NFL concussion case and was now versed in CTE. The difference for him was that he was a current player in the NFL and the case was only applicable to retired players. The hits that rang his bell for so many years were not part of the lawsuit. He, along with hundreds of other current players, was left out. All because the case had been exposed before he entered the NFL.

The explanation he received for not being able to join the lawsuit was something called assumption of risk. When he got drafted into the NFL, concussions and long-term injury were already in the news, so the League said he was fully aware of what he was getting himself into. Unfortunately for Matt, his symptoms were beginning. The rage, impulsivity, fading memory, and depression had taken over his existence.

His thoughts went back to the game. The whistle blew. He launched forward, colliding with the man opposite him, two bodies crashing like tectonic plates. Pain shot through his skull. Rage simmered beneath the helmet. The play ended, the crowd cheered, and the cycle reset.

Back in the suite, Bridgette sat quietly as the game wound down. Her secret—exposed just enough to share the weight—settled between her and Kelly like a stone.

No one else noticed. The wives clapped, the kids chanted, the game carried on.

Behind closed doors, though, another kind of game was being played—one where silence was the strategy, shamc was the defense, and survival was the only win.

And for Bridgette, the end of the fourth quarter didn't mean relief. It meant the longest part of the day was about to begin.

She followed the stream of families through the stadium corridor, past framed photos of legends frozen mid-stride. Down on the field, fireworks coughed smoke that drifted up like fog into the rafters. The elevator to the garage was filled with polite laughter, perfume, the chipper tone people use when they're speaking over something they don't want to name. Kelly kept a hand lightly on Bridgette's elbow. Neither of them spoke.

In the players' lot, engines turned over one by one. Security waved SUVs forward with the choreography of a parade. Bridgette slid behind the wheel and stared at her reflection in the rearview mirror: the sunglasses, the sleeve tugged down, the practiced smile. She reached back and touched the booster seat, then the little sock that had wriggled free and lay curled on the floor mat like a question mark. She drove home on autopilot, the highway a gray ribbon, the stadium shrinking behind her like a secret you can't un-tell.

The house was quiet when she walked in. She put her purse down carefully, the way you set something fragile on a table that might not hold. She checked the back door, locked it. She breathed.

An hour later, the garage door rumbled. The dogs barked and then went silent. Matt came in heavy, the way men walk when the game hasn't left their body yet. He kissed the air near her cheek and missed.

"Did you see that fourth-and-one?" he asked, already replaying the day on a loop, already bracing for the phantom hit he'd feel when he lay down.

She nodded. "I saw."

He opened a cabinet, then slammed it because it stuck. "Why's everything always in the wrong place?" he said, too loud for a kitchen.

"It's the same place," she answered softly. "It's always been the same place."

Something in him tightened. The rage flickered, then caught.

"Don't correct me," he said. But it wasn't the words. It was that far-off look that made her slide her hand along the counter until her fingers found the phone.

"I'm not," she whispered. "I'm just . . . here."

He stood there breathing, shoulders heaving, a mountain looking for someplace to fall. Then he turned and went down the hall. A door closed. A chair scraped. The house settled back into its careful stillness.

Bridgette stepped into the bathroom and locked the door. She lifted her sleeve again and studied the bruise in the bright light. It was angrier now, a bloom of storm over bone. She pressed her fingers to the edge and winced, then pressed harder, as if she could move the pain somewhere else.

Her phone buzzed. Kelly.

You okay?

Bridgette typed, I don't know. She erased it. She typed again, I'm scared he'll find out. Erased that too.

Kelly replied: I have a number. From a friend. Someone who helps. It's not the team.

There was a pause, three dots, a vanishing, three dots again.

You won't be alone if you call. He's with Boston University's brain lab. He may be able to help.

Bridgette stared at the screen until it went dark. In the mirror, the woman looking back at her didn't seem like someone who needed permission. She seemed like someone who needed a door that opened and stayed open.

From the hallway, the television came on. Highlights, talking heads, the soundtrack of denial wrapped in analysis. Great win. Gritty performance. This line is nasty. She turned the water on and tried to let the sound of the faucet drown out the noise.

The next morning wasn't better. Game film replaced highlights. The house hummed with subtle alarms—small misplacements, sentences left mid-clause, a temper that moved like weather across an open plain. She drove the kids to school and watched them walk in with their backpacks bumping against their shoulders, brave like only children can be. On the way back, she pulled into a Walmart lot and parked beneath the lone oak that grew from a square of stubborn dirt. She sat with both hands on the wheel and fought the urge to keep driving until the road ran out.

Her phone lit up again. Kelly. Did you call?

Bridgette typed, Not yet. She erased it. I heard he is a good man, Kelly wrote.

Bridgette copied the number she had been given into a new message and stared at the blank screen. The cursor blinked like a heart monitor. She didn't type. Instead, she scrolled through photos: Matt holding the baby in the hospital, Matt grilling in the backyard wearing a paper crown the kids made, Matt smiling half a smile after the Pro Bowl, helmet tucked under his arm like a promise. She closed the photo roll and opened the message again.

My name is Bridgette, she wrote. I need help.

She didn't send it. Not yet. She left the parking lot, turned onto the feeder road, and merged into traffic. Halfway home, a black SUV hugged her bumper too close, then swung into the next lane. She wasn't sure if it was coincidence or message. In this town, it could be both.

At home, the mailbox held a thick envelope with the team logo in the corner. She carried it inside and set it on the counter without opening it. When Matt came into the kitchen, he saw it, frowned, and slid it into a drawer.

"I'll handle that," he said, and closed the drawer like a vault.

Two nights later, a team "family coordinator" called to "check in." Her voice was honeyed, her questions careful. "Just making sure you're getting everything you need from us," she said. "We have resources." Bridgette almost laughed.

"What kind of resources?" she asked.

The coordinator spoke in spirals: counseling that came with forms, hotlines that reported to departments, support that felt like surveillance.

"We're fine," Bridgette said, and hung up.

She wasn't fine. She was awake at 5 a.m., scrolling through articles she had avoided for years, because sometimes loving someone means looking away just to keep loving them. But she didn't look away now. She found words she'd only heard in whispers and finally let them echo inside her head: concussion . . . CTE . . . mood regulation . . . impulse control . . . degeneration. She read the line twice that said, It's not you. It's the disease. The sentence cracked something open inside her—and didn't fix a thing.

She looked back at the text she'd drafted: My name is Bridgette. I need help. She hit send.

The next game came and went. The bruise on her arm faded from blue to green, then to yellow. Another appeared days later, smaller, maybe accidental—but patterns are just collections of small things pretending not to be connected. Kelly kept texting. Bridgette kept not answering.

After Thursday practice, Matt came home glassy-eyed and restless. He paced the hallway, stood in the doorway of the kids' room staring at the glow-in-the-dark stars on the ceiling like they might rearrange themselves into an answer. When Bridgette asked if he wanted to talk, he shook his head until his jaw clicked.

"About what?" he said. "There's nothing wrong."

That night, after the house fell silent, she checked her phone again. Still no reply from Chris, the brain specialist in Boston. Her finger hovered over the screen. The bedroom door creaked. Little feet padded across the hall. Her daughter stood in the doorway, hair tangled, cheeks flushed with sleep.

"Mom?" she whispered. "Is Daddy mad?"

Bridgette swallowed, forced a smile, shook her head. "No, baby. Daddy's just tired." She tucked her back in, smoothed the blanket, kissed her forehead.

When she returned to the kitchen, the phone was where she'd left it. The cursor blinked, steady as a clock, counting down a song she didn't want to sing alone. She didn't know that Chris would write back soon—that he was already overwhelmed, adding more names to the whiteboard in his office.

The next morning, Bridgette woke up when it was still dark outside. She stared at her phone, praying Chris could explain why the man she loved was no longer the man she had married.

A short time later, the phone buzzed once.

This is Chris. Tell me what's happening.

Bridgette got out of bed and looked down the hallway toward her children's rooms. Then back at the screen. Her thumbs hovered.

In the driveway, a car slowed as it rolled past, headlights sweeping across the blinds. The porch light flicked on, a motion sensor catching something in the dark. A neighbor's dog barked twice, then went silent.

She began to type: I heard you write names.

Three dots appeared. Paused. Disappeared. Appeared again. Like a heart trying to decide whether to beat.

And then they stopped. Silence so heavy that she felt like she couldn't breathe. Still not knowing what the whiteboard meant, she wondered whether one day Matt's name would be written along with the others.

10

THE KITCHEN

IN HOMES ACROSS AMERICA: 2015

There's something about a kitchen.

I'D been to a lot of homes since I started traveling. Each one different in geography, but the same in spirit. Men who had been heroes to strangers, sitting in their own homes, surrounded by the people who loved them, trying to make sense of what was happening to them.

One of the first homes I ever visited was that of Jim and Betty LeClair.

Jim was in his late fifties then, tall and polished, with the kind of posture that still hinted at the athlete he once was. If you didn't know, you might not notice anything wrong at first. He was charming, quick to smile, polite to a fault. But if you stayed long enough—if the conversation wandered a bit, if the details stretched beyond a couple of minutes—the mask began to slip. Memory doesn't lie, and it doesn't forgive.

Betty had been caring for Jim since his Alzheimer's diagnosis in February of 2014. She was one of those people whose gentleness could fill a room, the kind of woman who radiated warmth even when she was exhausted. Morning, noon, and night, she watched over him. Every movement, every forgotten word, every confused glance—she met it with patience.

The LeClair house was neat and full of light. Family photos lined the hallway. There was laughter in those frames—children's birthdays, holidays, barbecues, the kind of moments that anchor a family. Betty told me how the house used to sound when their kids were young, how Jim would come home from practice, scoop them up, and chase them around the living room. The laughter had faded over the years. Friends still came by now and then, but not like before. People didn't know what to say anymore.

When I sat with Jim at their kitchen table, he poured us each a cup of coffee. He told me stories that looped halfway through, moments that bled into each other. Sometimes he'd stop mid-sentence and stare at the wall, then smile like nothing had happened. Betty would finish the sentence for him, gently, like she'd done a hundred times before.

Jim didn't complain. He didn't curse fate or ask for pity. He just seemed confused by what was happening to him—like someone who had misplaced his own life and couldn't figure out where he'd left it.

The first time I visited, we talked for about two hours. The second time, I brought a small film crew. Chris O'Malley had asked me to travel with some photographers who were putting together a short video to present to the court—something to help show the human side of what we were fighting for. I chose Jim and Betty LeClair because they represented everyone else I'd met. Their story was everyone's story.

The camera captured what words could not: Betty's soft touch on Jim's arm when he lost his train of thought; the way she smiled through tears as she told me, "He still remembers our song—just not always my name."

I remember leaving their home that night and sitting in my rental car for a long time before driving away. The dashboard lights glowed faintly against the darkness outside. I thought about how unfair it all was—how many people like Jim and Betty were out there, fighting the same silent battle in houses just like theirs. The thought stayed with me. It still does.

Jim passed in November of 2019. He was sixty-nine years old. Betty was his high school sweetheart and the two were married in 1970. She lives alone now at their lake house. The home still shines with Jim's memories. I'm sure it always will.

From kitchen to kitchen, I traveled the country. Most of the men I visited had their wives or children present, but Roc's home was different. We sat alone, just the two of us, talking at the round wooden table in his kitchen.

Roc was in his mid-thirties—too young to be living the life he was living. Unlike Jim, Roc didn't have a Betty. He was single. No wife, no family. No one to check if he'd eaten or to remind him to take his medication. He lived alone in a small home that had once been filled with friends but now mostly echoed.

"I've been trying my best to get by, but that's about all I can do," Roc said.

As we spoke, I explained the settlement terms to him and told him how important it was for the players to understand and give a thumbs-up to the deal. He asked a few questions, quiet and thoughtful. Then he said something I'll always remember: "The hardest part isn't the pain or the forgetfulness—it's the loneliness."

"I just want to know someone's there," he said. "That if I forget who I am, somebody else will still know."

When I first met Roc, he was thirty-four. Still young enough to believe that promises meant something. He had faith the League would keep its word and compensate the players like I told him they would—that after everything he had given, fairness would find its way back to him. He wasn't bitter, and he wasn't asking for much. He didn't want revenge or riches—just enough to live, to know he'd have care when he could no longer care for himself. He wasn't asking for miracles. Only dignity.

The problem was that Roc never had the means to get a formal diagnosis. Without that qualifying condition, a financial payout was impossible. As part of the settlement, every player was entitled to one medical exam: a baseline assessment—the Baseline Assessment Program, or BAP for short. On paper, it sounded fair. In practice, it was anything but.

Before a physician could participate, they had to be vetted and approved by the NFL. That small detail didn't come to light until after the settlement was finalized and the program began. I'd call that a pretty important fact to mention up front, wouldn't you? Those same doctors were also paid by the League and required to follow the settlement's definitions of dementia—definitions far stricter than what most physicians in the real world would ever use.

Under the settlement agreement, in order to submit a claim, Roc would have to be examined by both a neurologist and a neuropsychologist. Both doctors would have to conclude that Roc had a qualifying dementia diagnosis. It didn't happen.

As far as I know, Roc still has not been able to resubmit a claim, and I'm sure he's still pushing for fairness. If I could wish one thing for him, it would be that his greatest fear of being left alone never comes true. I'm sure that he's still fighting for what he believes is right; I just hope that he is not fighting alone.

When I traveled south to visit another retired player suffering from Alzheimer's disease, his kitchen was heavy with a different kind of presence—sadness. The oven hummed softly, the smell of something baking filling the air as if the house itself was trying to pretend that everything was still normal, that life inside those walls hadn't quietly come apart.

He sat across from me at the table, a man still built like he could strap on pads and play another down. From the outside, you'd think he had everything—a beautiful wife, a nice home, grown children, and good friends. But inside, he was slipping away. The weight of his depression packed the room like humidity before a storm. Every question I asked felt like pulling teeth; every answer came slow, distant, hollowed out.

At one point, he got up to use the bathroom, and in the few minutes he was gone, his wife leaned across the table. Her voice trembled as she whispered, "Please, do whatever you can to get him some help. He talks about taking his own life." She told me she had found his gun a few days earlier out in the open and immediately hid it, terrified of what might happen if she left it alone. She wasn't crying, but her hands shook as she spoke—the kind of tremor that comes from living too long with fear.

When he returned, I asked if we could speak alone. I didn't want to betray her confidence, but I couldn't leave without addressing what she'd told me. I asked if the thoughts were real. He looked down for a long moment before nodding.

"Yeah," he said quietly. "They're real."

I told him how much he still had to live for—that he was a stand-up guy and a good human being. I told him about the other players I'd met, how the darkness had crept into their lives too, how they were fighting and how he was not alone, even when it felt that way. I don't know if my words helped, but I hoped they reached something inside him that the rest of us couldn't see.

He eventually received his approval letter from the claim administrator and a financial award for mild to moderate dementia. The money helped his family and gave them some measure of stability. But it didn't erase the sadness. It didn't fix the silence in that kitchen or the emptiness that followed him through the house. It just made life a little easier for the people he loved.

The images of those kitchens stayed with me. Every single one of them. The walls were different, the photographs and magnets were different, but the feeling was always the same. That's where the truth lived. Not in the legal briefs or the press releases, not in the promises made under oath—it lived across those tables, over cups of coffee that went cold while stories poured out.

It was in the way Betty LeClair's hand hovered just behind Jim's shoulder, ready to steady him if he stumbled. In the sound of her voice when she told me how he sometimes forgot her name but never forgot her face. It was in the way Roc stared down, trying to make sense of a language that made his life sound like a technicality. It was in the way the retired player's wife gripped her coffee cup like a lifeline, while the man she loved sat in the next room fighting battles no one could see.

I was the outsider. Not in a way that made me unwelcome, but in the sense that I was the one who could leave. I could shake hands, gather my notes, and drive away. They couldn't. Their world was that house, that kitchen, those walls closing in.

The real battle was fought here, in these kitchens, by families who had no choice but to keep showing up every day, even when hope was wearing thin. The court could argue over definitions and deadlines, but these people were living the consequences.

Sometimes, late at night, I still think about them—Jim and Betty, Roc, and the others whose names blur together now, but whose faces I'll never forget. I wonder how many of them are still out there waiting, still believing that fairness will find them.

Those kitchens were the front lines of a war no one televised—a quiet, relentless war waged in homes across the country. The league might have called it a settlement. I called it surrender—not by the players, but by the system that was supposed to protect them.

And yet, in every house, I saw something the system could never take away: love, loyalty, and the kind of devotion that doesn't care about definitions or awards or checks that never arrive. That's what stays with me. That's what defines real justice verses just an illusion of justice.

11

THE BANKER

PHILADELPHIA, FEDERAL DISTRICT COURT: 2018

Bankers and politicians.

I ONCE said that people are either bankers or politicians—driven by money or by power. Most are a blend of both. Money buys access; power decides how it's spent. Together, they run the world. In the NFL case, they ran everything.

The case took only a couple of years to win preliminary approval, but years passed before settlement money reached the players—some of them. Each day blurred into the next, and as months turned into seasons, desperation began to take hold. The men who had once dominated stadiums now struggled to hold their lives together. Their minds were unraveling faster than their finances, and every delay deepened both the confusion and the fear.

For their families, it was agony—watching the decline, the bills piling up, the hope fading. Desperation has a scent, and once it's in the air, the predators start to circle.

It started quietly—with a new breed of predator. They called themselves "litigation funders," and they arrived in tailored suits carrying the language of salvation. They'd never stepped onto a field or taken a hit, but they knew how to spot weakness. They could smell desperation and knew exactly how to sell hope to the hopeless.

They came for the players—and for me.

I represented the men they wanted to reach. My access, my trust with the players—that was their way in. I was the bridge, and they were eager to cross it.

Some could barely hold a conversation. Some forgot their children's names. But all of them shared the same problem: The settlement process was moving at the speed of bureaucracy, and their bills were coming fast. To many men ruled by confusion and pain, they sounded like salvation.

"Why wait?" they asked, leaning forward with rehearsed empathy. "We can get you cash now. You've earned it."

The men nodded. They needed money for their mortgages, their medicine, their children's tuition. Fast money was better than distant promises. They signed the papers.

What they didn't understand—what no one had explained to them—was that these weren't loans. They were sales. The funders weren't offering help; they were buying the players' rights to future settlement claims. For every $1 thousand advanced, the funders claimed thousands more from settlements that hadn't even been paid yet.

By the time the players realized the truth, the ink was dry. Their signatures had sold away what little stability they had left.

When Judge Brody found out what was happening, she called for an emergency hearing. O'Malley led the crusade. The courtroom was thick with tension and fluorescent light. On one side, retired players once cheered by millions now sat quietly, their wives holding folders of medical reports, deceptive funding agreements, and, most of all, half-truths. Across from them sat the funders and their lawyers—men in crisp suits hiding behind the letter of the law.

The judge didn't need long to see what had been done. The contracts were one-sided, deceptive, written to exploit men who could no longer comprehend the fine print. She called it what it was—"exploitation by predators." One by one, she voided the deals. Every contract with a player. Every "advance." Every dollar taken in deceit.

For a moment, justice actually worked. The courtroom exhaled.

The players, for once, were freed from the wolves that had come to feed on their injuries.

Several weeks later, Chris O'Malley, the man spearheading the opposition to these vultures, asked me for a favor.

"Craig," he said, "I want you to meet someone. He's a friend of mine. He's not like the other funders. He's with a bank—The Lawyer's Bank. They're trying to help the players who can't afford to wait. Fair deals. Compassionate terms. No predators here. You know these families. You understand what they're going through. Sit down with the bank president, he's my good friend. Explain the settlement process. Help him figure out how to make this work."

His tone was casual. I wanted to believe it. I thought I was being asked to help craft something ethical—a fair bridge for struggling men who had already lost too much.

So, I agreed to meet.

The bank's president, Morris, arrived confident, polished, perfectly rehearsed. He listened carefully, nodding at all the right moments, his pen moving with quiet precision as he took notes. He wanted to know everything: how the claims process worked, how long it dragged on, how desperate the families had become. And then his questions turned clinical—focused on recovery amounts, projections, probabilities.

I explained that compensation was calculated using a grid—a matrix that weighed how long a player had been in the League as well as his age at the time of diagnosis. Morris leaned back in his chair, eyes sharp behind the smile. "Then let's develop a formula," he said. "Something that predicts what each player might recover. That way, I can get their families as much money as possible now—relieve some of the immediate pressure."

Strategic compassion dressed as finance. Across the table, Morris's associates chimed in with their own questions, their tone polite but probing, dissecting every detail of the settlement as if they were studying for an exam.

And all the while, a quiet thought kept scratching at the back of my mind:

If O'Malley and Morris were such close friends, why hadn't O'Malley just met with him himself? He was the one who'd negotiated the entire settlement—the architect of the grid we were now dissecting.

I didn't have the answer then. But when I finally learned it, it explained everything.

Together, Morris and his associates discussed what I thought was a framework to protect the players—a formula to keep predatory terms out of the equation. I thought I was helping build a bridge. What I didn't know was that I was handing them a map—a detailed map of the settlement and a forecast of the anticipated payouts.

Weeks later, I saw the formula. Clean, efficient, predatory. A machine built to calculate risk, assign value, and determine exactly how much of a man's future could be bought for cash today. It was math masquerading as mercy.

This wasn't about helping players. It was about profit.

And suddenly, I understood why O'Malley hadn't sat at that table himself. Why he'd sent me instead.

Because he couldn't be seen there. Because he had something to hide.

He had previously sat on the Bank's Board of Directors—the very institution whose president I'd just helped arm with inside knowledge of the settlement process. And from what I later learned, he still held shares in that bank.

A monumental conflict of interest.

He'd disclosed it to no one.

While he stood in front of the judge condemning funders as predators, he was quietly tethered to a bank poised to profit from the very same predation. And by using me—my credibility, my relationships, my good faith—he gave his arrangement legitimacy.

It wasn't an accident. It was strategy. And by introducing me to Morris, he hadn't just used me, he jeopardized my very involvement in the case.

For O'Malley, that kind of conflict wasn't just unethical—it was disqualifying, at least if the court ever found out. In any other case, it would have cost him his position as lead counsel. But in this one, there wasn't even a whisper, because the information wasn't public and the court had no idea who the Bank was, let alone O'Malley's connection to the financial institution.

But silence never lasts forever—not when truth is pushing from beneath it.

Several months later, Gene Rockman filed a motion asking for balance, not overthrow. His motion sought to have his firm appointed to work alongside O'Malley—not beneath him. It was a simple idea, really: two leaders instead of one unchecked authority. A safeguard. A shared responsibility.

Rockman argued that the players—the men whose lives were unraveling while others profited from their pain—deserved accountability at the top. They needed someone to make sure no single lawyer held all the power, all the access, all the control.

He was right, and I knew it.

So I supported the motion. Not out of politics, but out of principle. Because I'd seen what happened when power went unchallenged—how easily it curdled into arrogance, how quickly it began to consume the very people it was meant to serve.

Supporting Rockman wasn't rebellion. It was conscience.

That was all it took. In O'Malley's world, my decision had to be punished.

Several weeks later, O'Malley's response to Rockman's motion was filed with the court. I read it carefully. Buried in the middle of it, like a dagger between the lines, was my name—and my firm. O'Malley accused me of soliciting players on behalf of litigation funders because I supported Rockman's joint leadership request.

An appartent effective lie. It didn't need proof, just doubt. It shifted attention away from him and toward me. The move was obviously pure vindictiveness—cold, precise, and intentional.

I didn't wait to respond. The next morning, I filed a declaration directly with Judge Brody. I laid it all out—that I never solicited players for any funding company. I told her it was really O'Malley who was soliciting for a funding company—the bank. I explained the introduction, the conflict of interest, the concealment, the formula Morris had developed, all at O'Malley's request. I attached the proof: the emails, the correspondence, the documentation. It was all there in black and white.

My filing was visible on the federal docket for fifteen minutes. Then it was gone. One word replaced it: SEALED.

When I called the clerk to find out who had sealed my filing, his answer came softly after several minutes on hold. "The judge."

That was the moment I realized that truth didn't matter. The system wasn't blind. It was complicit.

I learned later that a local reporter from down south had happened to check the docket during the fifteen minutes that the filing was visible. She downloaded it, read it, figured it was important, and sent it to ESPN. Within days, headlines blazed: Documents allege lead attorney in NFL concussion deal failed to disclose conflict of interest.

For forty-eight hours, it felt like light had finally found its way into the dark. The story was published online and appeared on-air. The Select Few were talking, whispering amongst one another. Reporters called. I thought, maybe this time, truth might outrun power.

But then the story vanished, and the court never addressed it. There was no hearing, no ruling, not even a question from the bench. In any other case, a conflict like that would have deto-nated a career. Here, it didn't even ripple the surface. The silence wasn't ignorance. It was intentional. The machine knew how to protect its own.

Deceit doesn't always announce itself with lies. Sometimes, it hides in the quiet—in the moments when people look away because the truth costs too much to acknowledge.

Betrayal isn't always loud. Sometimes it's procedural. It lives in sealed orders and redacted paragraphs.

Vindictiveness has its own rhythm. It doesn't roar; it waits. It waits until your guard is down, until you've convinced yourself you're fighting on the same side, and then it reminds you that power has no allies—only instruments.

That's what this was. A warning dressed as procedure. A silencing disguised as professionalism.

But the story didn't end there. What began as betrayal bled into something darker. I began to understand how the system feeds itself—how every deal, every sealed filing, every whisper of "procedure" hides a pulse of profit beneath it.

The same funders who had preyed on the players also came for me. Years into the fight, drained of cases, buried in debt from uncompensated work, I was vulnerable—just like the men I'd tried to protect. One of the funding agents called, smooth-voiced, promising relief. "Craig," he said, "you've earned this. You are owed millions in common benefit monies. Let us help you bridge the gap. There's absolutely no risk to you."

I told myself I was keeping the lights on, keeping the mission alive. But the moment I signed, I had become what I feared most—another man caught in the illusion of control while someone else counted the cost.

When the repayments came due, I realized I'd walked straight into their trap. The numbers didn't add up and the hundreds of thousands of dollars I had already repaid them went mostly to "transaction fees." They were going to do whatever was necessary to get their money, along with the interest they claimed the deal carried. I'd been fooled, used, and discarded in the very same machine I had once fought to dismantle.

I lost my savings, including the money I had put away for my children's college tuitions, along with my retirement.

And that's when I understood the cruel symmetry of it all—the game was never about justice. It was about leverage.

Money doesn't need to shout. It whispers. It seduces. It convinces you that it's salvation until the moment you realize it was the devil all along.

That's what this chapter of my life taught me—that the devil doesn't arrive with horns and fire. He arrives in cufflinks and good lighting. He calls you by your first name. He tells you he's your friend. And he makes you believe it.

The court could seal my words. The headlines could fade. But no gavel can erase the truth: Money corrupted everything it touched. It bought loyalty. It bought silence. And in the end, it bought me, too—just long enough to make me believe I was winning.

I still think about those players—kitchens smelling of coffee and fear, wives holding folders they didn't understand, men who trusted the wrong people because hope was all they had.

They were the ones who deserved better. We all did.

And maybe that's what hell really is—not fire, not brimstone, but silence. The silence of knowing that everyone who could have spoken, didn't. The silence of truth buried beneath wealth and ego.

Because sometimes, money isn't the root of evil. It is evil.

And the devil doesn't come to take your soul. He comes to buy it.

As for what came next—the silence would grow louder.

What began in courtrooms and contracts would test not only what I believed in, but who I was.

12

FINAL APPROVAL

PHILADELPHIA, FEDERAL DISTRICT COURT: SPRING 2015

The illusion of justice.

SUPPORTERS of the settlement made a fair argument: Centralized relief promised speed, certainty, and an end to years of litigation. Families wouldn't have to prove a league-wide cover-up in court; instead, they'd receive a clear pathway to compensation and testing. That promise could have been true—if the rules hadn't concentrated discretion behind closed doors, if "neutral" procedures hadn't become hurdles, and if the men most affected hadn't been asked to trade their voices for finality.

The courthouse that morning pulsed like a stadium before kickoff. The air was damp with rain on wool coats, burned coffee from the lobby kiosk, and the tang of ink and sweat. Security guards herded people through metal detectors in long, impatient lines. Reporters clustered in the hallway, adjusting tripods and batteries, voices hushed but urgent. The marble floors amplified every sound: heels clicking, canes tapping, shoes scuffing as spectators pressed toward the chamber doors.

The players arrived slowly, deliberately, wives guiding them down aisles and into rows. Some carried themselves with rigid dignity, jaw clenched against the tremor in their hands. Others stumbled slightly, not entirely sure where they were. A few wore their old team blazers, sleeves now too tight on bodies that had swollen with medication or sagged with illness. Their presence was an indictment before a single word was spoken—living evidence of what the game had taken and refused to give back. Their wives hovered close, one with a hand pressed constantly against her husband's back, another whispering directions he could no longer remember.

This wasn't just a hearing. It was a trial of hope itself.

The clerk's voice boomed: "All rise."

The scrape of benches, the shuffling of shoes, the rustle of fabric—it all collided as the room surged upward. Judge Anita Brody stepped through the door and mounted the bench. She looked small behind the wood, almost fragile in her black robe, but her presence was undeniable. The silence that fell was immediate and absolute.

"Good morning, everyone. Please have a seat."

The room shifted back into stillness: the creak of jackets, the hiss of skirts across benches, the muted cough of someone trying too hard to hide it. Behind me, a wife whispered a prayer into her hand, her lips barely moving. Another smoothed her husband's tie and dabbed his forehead with a tissue. The air itself seemed to hold its breath.

Chris O'Malley rose first. He buttoned his jacket, smoothed his lapel, and walked to the lectern with the careful gravity of a man who knew the room was his. Every step was deliberate, every gesture calculated. He adjusted the microphone, cleared his throat softly, and began.

For half an hour, he spoke. Less a legal argument than a performance. His cadence rose and fell like a sermon, pauses dropped at just the right moments, eyes lifted skyward when words like "justice" or "duty" fell from his lips. His hands carved the air like a conductor's baton, shaping the silence as much as the words.

He spoke of fairness. He spoke of closure. He spoke of the suffering of the men behind him, their sacrifice, their need for relief. He invoked inevitability, justice, duty.

He looked at Judge Brody, at the reporters, at the wives whose eyes glistened in the gallery. It was a show, and he performed it well.

And then, at the precise moment, he unveiled the crescendo he'd been building toward:

"Your Honor, there is one reason above all others that warrants this settlement being made final. One reason that speaks louder than any legal brief or expert testimony: ninety-nine-point-one percent of the retired player population has endorsed this deal. Ninety-nine-point-one percent. That is unheard of."

O'Malley sat down, expression smooth, as though history itself had just been drafted in his name.

Then Brad Karp, representing the Laegue rose. Polished, cold, the embodiment of Wall Street power. His voice was steady, clipped, almost dismissive of the theater that had come before.

“Judge,” he said with the faintest smile, “Mr. O’Malley said it all. Ninety-nine-point-one percent approval. That number alone tells you everything you need to know.”

The echo cut deeper than the original.

He let it hang.

The number was a weapon. The number was a shield. It was both sword and sanctuary.

And it was mine.

I sat there listening, my mind spinning back through the years: red-eye flights across the country, shoulders aching from hours in cheap seats; banquet halls full of broken men clutching my arm after speeches; kitchen tables where wives whispered their fear that their husbands might not wake in the morning; alumni chapter meetings where former teammates clapped me on the back and said “brother,” trusting me with their futures.

I remembered the tears, the anger, the despair. I remembered the woman who told me she’d hidden the guns.

I had carried the burden of persuasion. I had stood in living rooms, explaining a settlement I hadn’t drafted. I gave voice to hope when the men in suits only offered fine print. Ninety-nine-point-one percent had trusted because I asked them to.

And now those words—the fruit of my sacrifice—rolled easily off the lips of O’Malley and Karp, trophies they claimed as their own.

The irony burned. Because what no one else in that courtroom yet knew—not the reporters scribbling furiously, not the wives clinging to their husbands, not even the players themselves—was that final approval wasn’t the finish line. It was the opening whistle. The rules had already been written, buried in fine print, tilted against the very men they were supposed to protect. Families would soon learn they'd have to fight for what they'd been promised, clawing through audits and denials.

The players thought they'd won. They had no idea the trap was already sprung.

And I was the one who'd walked them into it.

Still, there was the carrot. The "common benefit fund." One hundred twelve million dollars set aside by the NFL, reserved for the handful of lawyers whose work had benefited the entire class. From the beginning I'd been told: five million, at least. Maybe more. Recognition. Acknowledgment that I'd carried the 99.1 percent.

But nothing was ever in writing. Nothing.

Once, early on, I'd made the mistake of sending O'Malley a text to confirm something. My phone rang instantly.

"Craig," his voice roared, "don't you ever put anything in writing. Don't you get it? Everything's discoverable. Nothing in writing, ever."

At the time, I believed him. I thought it was strategy. I thought it was about shielding us from the NFL's lawyers. What I didn't see was that it was about control. Without paper, without proof, without anything binding, O'Malley alone would decide what my sacrifice was worth.

Years before final approval, a litigation funder had approached me. He spoke with the smoothness of a man who'd rehearsed the same pitch a thousand times.

"Craig, take a couple million now. Use it for travel, outreach, education. Build websites, produce videos. You'll repay it when the fees come in, and you'll still walk away with millions. No risk. None."

He was convincing. Too convincing. I believed him. I took the money. I spent it on the work—on the flights, the hotel rooms, the brochures, the endless circuit of city after city, building that 99.1 percent.

O'Malley knew. He always knew. But he didn't care. Because in the end, O'Malley was going to do what O'Malley was going to do.

The day in court rolled forward like a train on rails. Objectors rose and spoke, voices quavering as they tried to pierce language designed to resist them. An epidemiologist droned about incidence and prevalence until the numbers blurred into rain on glass. A neurologist said "degeneration" and someone two rows behind me bit down on their knuckle until it bled.

Reporters scribbled until their fingers cramped. Marshals refilled carafes. The fluorescent lights hummed like cicadas.

And then the gavel.

One sharp knock several weeks later that stamped the future.

Approval.

O'Malley shook Karp's hand, smiling like a man who knew exactly which door led to the counting room. Wives clutched one another and caught up on things. Players nodded solemnly, some aware, others unaware.

In the hallway, microphones swarmed O'Malley first.

"How does it feel?" one reporter asked.

"Historic," he said. "Fair."

He said fair the way a magician says abracadabra. The word made the trick work.

I slipped out the side doors into the cold of Market Street. Sirens wailed in the distance. The bell in the tower chimed the hour, and I counted anyway, because I needed to hear it for myself.

My phone buzzed. A text from the funder: Clock has started. Expecting allocation soon?

Another buzz. An email from O'Malley's office: Common benefit fee declaration submissions due.

A document from the court with a line that mattered more than any other:

Lead counsel is authorized to allocate common benefit fees.

That night, at home with my family, I spread papers across the desk—declarations, travel logs, billable hours, the letters I'd received from high-profile players attesting to my influence in the lawsuit and settlement from start to finish.

Over the next several weeks, I drafted my submission. I listed the cities, the meetings, the endorsements. I laid out the 99.1 percent. I wrote in the system's language—dates, miles, names, outcomes—and I attached every scrap of evidence I still had.

Midnight. Send.

Morning: silence.

I was awarded less than $1 million—not enough to cover what I owed the litigation funder. A nominal amount. A token gesture. A pat on the head for the outsider who'd carried the weight but would never be welcomed into the club.

That was the price of being the outsider. That was the cost of not belonging to the Select Few.

Ninety-nine-point-one percent was mine. But the rewards never would be.

I closed the order and stared at my reflection in the black glass of the TV in my office.

Somewhere in the city, champagne corks were popping. Somewhere else, a widow was filling out yet another form.

The office felt warmer than normal. The future felt narrower. I thought of every living room I'd stood in, every promise I'd made, and the one promise I believed most: that the people who did the work would be compensated fairly.

I thought the gavel's echo would mean closure, but it only sharpened the sound of doors slamming shut. Approval had been stamped into law, but justice had been bartered away in the process. The settlement was final, yet nothing felt finished. The promises I'd carried across the country, the voices I'd sworn to protect, now hung in the balance of a system designed to deny them.

And as I sat there with the court order in my hands, I knew the real battle hadn't ended in Judge Brody's courtroom.

It had only just begun.

13

THE RELEASE

RICHMOND, VIRGINIA: WINTER 2018

The silence became permanent.

WINTER seeped into the seams—through warped window frames, under shifting doors, into corners where baseboards pulled away from drywall.

She knew this house's sounds the way a nurse knows a ward at night: the vent's tick when heat kicked on, the gulp of the kitchen pipes after the toilet filled, the refrigerator's drone that consumed midnight's quiet. Some nights she'd lie there, counting seconds between furnace cycles, willing time to keep going.

There'd been laughter here. A scuffed hallway line marked where daughters bounced and ran toward the kitchen. Pencil marks by the pantry door tracked growth—dates, initials, each line higher than the last. A note on the fridge said REMEMBER

MILK, the heart smeared by a small thumb, pointing both forward and back like a map of everything that followed.

The league would call this the human cost in a press release, if they called it anything. She had no such words. She had grocery lists, calendars, test result folders. She had survival strategies: cheap cereal that stayed crunchy, laundry done Sunday night before the energy company cut power, gas bought ten dollars at a time to maintain an illusion of control.

She had faith, though it'd changed shape. It used to look like Sunday morning. Now it looked like getting out of bed when the alarm was just memory.

No one told her courage sounded like quiet. That it could be the softest thing in the room and still be the strongest.

Downstairs, the TV cast blue light without sound. The chair that belonged to him faced it at an angle, as if the body still remembered how to find the best line to the screen even if the mind didn't. The remote had been taped together twice—electrician's tape first, then clear packing tape when the first layer peeled and collected lint. The batteries lived in a ceramic bowl on the coffee table, mixed with pennies, a church key, a rusted screw no one remembered removing. She'd put them there because losing the batteries felt like losing control of the only machine she could still operate. It made the house feel obedient for five seconds at a time.

Before the lawyer called, she'd already done the math she'd promised herself she'd never do. A month of mortgage, two of utilities, groceries pared to staples. The girls had asked about field trip fees and she'd said, "We'll see," which everyone knows means no.

She'd sold the last ring she swore she'd keep, the one with the nick you could only feel when the stone turned just right.

Sometimes she'd rub the empty place, believing you could miss a thing so hard the skin learned it.

She'd once believed love would protect them. That loving a man like him—capable, faithful, built for hard things—was its own armor. He'd been the one who carried the heavy end of the couch when they moved, who lifted sleeping children from the backseat without waking them, who could deadlift an engine block and then hold a newborn without bending her wrist. Love wasn't armor, she understood now. Love was the reason you walked into the fire.

Upstairs, footsteps crossed and paused. The girls whispered the way people whisper in hospitals, a hush edged with worry. She could tell which was which by cadence. The oldest was careful with words, the middle one stacked sentences then knocked them over with a joke, the youngest had a breathless way of speaking that made everything sound urgent. They'd learned to move like weather—fast when they had to be, soft when the air demanded it, always watching the horizon of a man's mood that the man himself could no longer read.

The email would arrive shortly, the lawyer had said. Fourteen pages. Simple. The sort of simple complicated people describe to those already standing on a cliff. She'd smiled into the phone and said thank you. She'd hung up and held the handset against her chest until the display light timed out. Then she'd wiped the fingerprint from the screen because fingerprints were proof someone still lived here.

On the mantel, his life existed in frames. Pop Warner with a helmet too big for his ears and a grin too big for the helmet. Draft night on a couch that sagged in the middle, cheap paneling behind him trying its best to look like wood. A sideline shot with sweat shining like varnish on his face and a smile that made her forgive every Thanksgiving missed for road games. A picture of him holding their smallest daughter with that careful, surprised expression men get when they learn strength can be used for gentleness. She didn't dust them anymore. Dust felt like a witness. To wipe it away would be to say time wasn't happening. But time was happening. It filled the room the way the refrigerator hum does, asking nothing and taking everything.

When the girls told friends their dad used to play football, the friends always asked the same question: "Was he famous?"

The girls would look at each other and one would say, "He's ours," as if that were the better answer.

She had a list of numbers taped inside the kitchen cabinet: the neurologist, the claims administrator, the case manager's assistant, the school nurse, the auto shop, the pastor. Under the list she'd written three words that used to feel like a plan and now felt like a dare:

MAKE IT THROUGH.

She wasn't sure when she'd stopped adding "TODAY" and started adding "AGAIN."

The cursor blinked on the laptop like a tiny lighthouse. She kept turning toward it to see if the email had arrived. The phone rang, rang again, then the inbox chimed.

The house was quiet, but not peaceful. Heavy, suffocating silence follows when words no longer matter. The refrigerator hummed its stubborn hymn. The television flickered in the corner, muted, light crawling across the living room walls. He sat in his recliner, massive shoulders still filling the chair, the frame of an athlete who'd once silenced stadiums with a single block.

But his eyes were glassy, distant, following nothing. He was fifty-seven and already half gone.

His wife waited to open the email. The screen's glow highlighted her clenched jaw, tight shoulders. She carried herself like a woman bracing for impact, though the impact had already happened years ago, long before the first doctor dared whisper the word dementia.

The children lingered on the stairs, whispering to each other in voices that carried a child's fear. They watched their father with sadness, confusion, and something they couldn't yet name—grief in its earliest form. The older one hushed the younger two with a trembling hand, then sat halfway down the steps as if moving closer might wake a monster they couldn't see.

The phone rang again. On speakerphone, the lawyer's voice filled the room, clinical and tired. "The claim form should be in your inbox. It's fourteen pages. I'll guide you through it."

Fourteen pages. The NFL called it "simple." To his wife, it was a mountain of paper designed not for justice but attrition.

Before she could open the email, the house phone rang. It was her cousin. She told the lawyer she needed a minute and answered, stepping into the kitchen. When she returned, her face had paled.

"It's about my grandmother," she told her husband gently, though his blank stare confirmed he didn't understand. "They're saying she wants to change her will."

The words sounded absurd in that living room—absurd and cruel. Her grandmother had developed Alzheimer's several years earlier. Any will she signed would be meaningless—no judge would accept it.

The law recognized what she couldn't do: She no longer had capacity to know what she was doing.

The irony struck like lightning. Because at that moment she opened the email, the NFL concussion claim form had arrived.

Fourteen pages of questions, attachments, medical records. A labyrinth disguised as a form. And on the very last page, the signature line.

His wife scrolled slowly, breath catching as she read the block of text starting on page thirteen and continuing onto page fourteen, looming above the signature line. It wasn't a sentence; it was a wall. A fortress of words constructed to bury truth. She whispered the language aloud, voice breaking:

"In consideration of the benefits included in the settlement agreement and operation of the final court order and judgment of the settlement agreement, I hereby waive, release, and discharge, and hold harmless the NFL and all of the NFL parties for any claim I may have in the past, present, or future, whether known or unknown, whether foreseen or unforeseen, relating to or in connection with concussions or head trauma. I specifically release the NFL for any condition I may have now or learn I have in the future involving CTE."

She gripped the table's edge, fingers tight. "How can he sign this? He doesn't even know what day it is. He doesn't know who the president is. How can this mean anything?"

On the other end, the lawyer's voice was quiet, almost apologetic. "I didn't write it. There's no negotiation. If he doesn't sign, there's no payout."

Her throat tightened. Her children stood frozen on the stairs. The man in the chair shifted, lost, unaware of the storm swirling around him. The dog raised its head, confused by the currents of a house that used to feel certain.

His wife knelt beside him, pressing the pen into his hand. His fingers curled weakly, trembling as he lowered the tip to the page. His eyes were vacant, his hand unsteady. Still, he scratched his name across the line. A signature without understanding. A release without consent. The ink looked too blue for something so final.

Somewhere in a New York office, the NFL had already won.

The form was filed. Then came the waiting for the decision. How much would he be compensated? Either way, no amount would compensate this man for his or his family's suffering. No amount.

Days bled into weeks. Weeks into months. She kept hope alive because what else was left? She told herself the check would come. That this suffering, this humiliation, would at least mean security for their children. She folded laundry she could barely afford to wash, stacked bills on the counter into small, neat towers like tiny city skylines of worry, and circled due dates on a wall calendar that never stopped whispering "late." Notices in the mailbox. Foreclosure of the family home was less than a year away. She lied to herself because the truth was unbearable.

Three months later, a single envelope arrived. Thin. Too thin. She knew before she opened it.

The letter inside was clinical, detached. Your claim has been reviewed. It has been denied. The administrator does not find it valid.

Her chest collapsed. The daughters cried. Even the lawyer's voice, when she called him, was empty, rehearsed: "I'm sorry. There's nothing more we can do, except appeal the decision. But to do that... the settlement administrator requires a payment of $1,000. It must come from the player."

His wife blinked. "What?"

"I'm sorry. It's in the settlement agreement. That's what was agreed to by Class Counsel. That's what the NFL demanded."

She stared down at her husband—eyes glazed over, mouth twitching slightly, a man locked behind glass. A man who couldn't remember what day it was, couldn't name his own children on a bad day, and still, somehow, the NFL required him to personally pay the fee to appeal a denial of benefits for the disease they'd caused.

Her voice was trembling, rising now. "So let me get this straight. He's too sick to remember how to get dressed some mornings, but he's well enough to be held legally and financially responsible for filing his own appeal?"

The lawyer didn't answer right away. A pause. A breath. Then, gently: "I didn't make the rules. But yes. That's how the settlement's structured. If the appeal isn't accompanied by the $1,000 payment, it's automatically rejected."

She nearly dropped the phone. Rage and helplessness crashed inside her like waves against steel. Upstairs, the girls had gathered outside their shared room, listening. They'd grown up with the sounds of football on TV, the pride in their father's name, the roar of crowds playing in their heads like fairy tales. And now—this.

Later that night, after a dinner none of them could eat, the girls called their mom into their room.

They sat cross-legged on the floor, the youngest already in tears.

"We'll get the money, Mom," said the oldest. "We'll figure it out."

Her lip quivered. "You shouldn't have to—"

"We want to," said the middle daughter. "He took care of us."

They pooled what they had. A few hundred in savings. A birthday gift check left unspent. The rest would come from selling things—an old bike, a laptop, tutoring shifts, waitressing tips. They'd make it happen. Somehow. The oldest wrote a list on a yellow pad. Sell: bike, guitar, extra TV. Extra shifts: Saturdays. Ask Aunt Kay? Hope is a muscle; they flexed it until it ached.

She kissed each of them, her heart both broken and full.

The appeal was filed the following week. The $1,000 wired. Another digital form submitted into the black hole of bureaucracy.

The lawyer called back with the steps. "The NFL has thirty days to file their response. Once that happens, the settlement claims administrator will issue a ruling."

"But the administrator works with the NFL," she said bitterly.

He hesitated. "They're... appointed under the terms of the agreement. They're supposed to be neutral."

She scoffed. She'd been married to a professional athlete for over twenty years. She knew what "supposed to" meant.

There was no real hope—only the shape of it, worn down like an old statue that still stood because no one had the heart to tear it down.

The waiting returned, heavier now. The days blurred. She took on more shifts at the hospital to keep occupied. And he—he stayed in that chair. Sometimes he'd smile at nothing. Sometimes he'd scream at shadows. Other times he'd rage, and fear would come over the family. The house learned to tiptoe around the hours when his temper arrived like weather—unpredicted, undeniable.

Once, she found him outside at dawn in his boxers, holding a planter like it was a football. He thought he was at training camp. He called a cadence to no one, planted his feet in the wet grass, and waited for a snap the sun refused to give him. She wrapped a blanket around his shoulders and led him inside while the neighbors' sprinklers whispered along the sidewalk like gossip.

A week later, the envelope came.

Thicker than the first.

But just as cruel.

Your appeal has been reviewed and denied. Final decision. No further action may be taken.

Her knees buckled. She sank to the floor, the letter in her lap like an autopsy report. Everything blurred. Her daughters' voices. Her husband humming a song he couldn't name. The clock ticking like a countdown to nothing.

She wept.

Two days passed. She didn't know what made her do it—maybe instinct, maybe prayer. She remembered something a teammate's wife had once said, years ago in passing, back when things were only starting to unravel.

"Call Craig. When everything else fails. Call Craig."

She found his number in an old group chat and dialed it.

He answered. "This is Craig."

She hesitated, then told him everything.

The denial. The appeal. The $1,000. The lies. The signature her husband didn't understand. The shotgun in the corner.

He was quiet for a moment.

Craig arrived the next morning in jeans and a windbreaker, boots still muddy from wherever he'd been before. He didn't bring a briefcase. He didn't need one. He stood on the porch and waited, like a man asking the house for permission to enter.

He didn't say much when he walked into the living room. Just looked around.

He looked at the stained carpet, the pile of unopened bills, the prescription bottles lining the counter—a family's biography written in paper and orange plastic.

Then he saw the man in the recliner. And he froze.

He walked over slowly, like approaching a fallen comrade.

"Hey, big man," Craig said softly.

No response.

Craig turned back to the wife.

He nodded toward the far corner, toward the weapon half-hidden under a blanket. "I think you should get that out of the house. Today."

She nodded, hands suddenly shaking. "He doesn't even remember it's there most days. But when he does... he just stares at it."

Craig didn't blink. "We've lost too many already."

She looked down, ashamed.

Then he laid out the truth. No sugar. No legalese. Just the hard steel of reality.

"Lead counsel negotiated and entered into this settlement agreement on behalf of all the players. That's the deal. That's the wall. Everything that's happening to you, it was baked in from day one. The judge? She rubber-stamps everything. You could bring her a hundred pages of evidence, and she'd still say no. Because that's how this is built. It's not about justice. It's about finality."

She sat on the couch's edge, head in her hands. "So there's nothing we can do."

Craig didn't answer right away.

Instead, he looked at the man in the chair again, watched his mouth twitch as he smiled at a baseball game from fifteen years ago, playing only in his mind. He noticed the framed photo on the mantle: a young lineman grinning through eye black, a toddler on his shoulders reaching for the sky like it was something you could grab if your father was tall enough.

Then he looked at the wife. At the tired, broken mother of three who'd carried the weight of silence for far too long.

"I'm so sorry. Never lose hope, because hope is what keeps all of us going."

Craig's words hung in the air like dust in a sunbeam.

She wanted to believe that. God, she wanted to believe it. And for a moment, it almost felt true.

But deep down, she knew the fight against the NFL and knew the odds.

Because beneath the flicker and the fury, she already knew what Craig hadn't said.

No one beats the NFL.

Not the players.

Not the families.

Not the truth.

This was a billion- machine dressed in America's colors, built on bodies, protected by lawyers, and cheered on by millions. It didn't matter how much sicker her husband became, or how many others fell with him. The headlines would fade. The settlement would stand. The game would go on.

They'd won.

The league had covered itself in legal armor and declared it a victory for all. And the fans? They'd keep cheering, filling stadiums with deafening roars, never hearing the silence echoing in homes like hers.

Because in this home, there was no cheering. No lights. No Sunday rituals.

Only the sound of a man lost in time.

Only the soft weeping of daughters trying to be brave.

Only the haunted quiet of a woman who'd done everything right—and still lost everything that mattered.

The silence wasn't just silence anymore.

It was a sentence.

It was suffocation.

Injustice, control imbalance, and despair disguised as silence.

Several years later, with hope having long disappeared since the denials, her phone rang.

It was Craig. He said hello and told her he was holding a folder. She could hear papers shuffling. Then silence.

"You need to read this," he whispered.

Inside the file were audit reports, internal memos, lines in tiny print—and the single phrase that strangled her heart: race-norming.

"They'd baked it into the settlement itself," Craig said, voice sad but firm. "The assumption that Black brains begin at a lower baseline than white ones. That when a Black player sat for cognitive tests, the bar to show 'decline' would be set higher—because the drafters of this billion-dollar machine secretly believed Black men were already broken."

Doctors were told to adjust scores downward. Claims denied—not because the brain was uninjured, but because the measurement was rigged. In effect, the League had paid less to Black survivors not because they were less harmed, but because the rules said they had less to lose.

She listened with intensity, shocked at what she was hearing. The words "conceal a lie" came out of her mouth unintentionally.

All this time she'd grieved, fought, pleaded—and the system had quietly, invisibly stacked the deck against them, masked beneath "neutral standards."

Craig's voice broke. "They called it science. They called it 'norms.' But it was prejudice in a lab coat. And they built it in from the start."

She could hear the tears in her voice and the fierce anger in her tone. How many others, she wondered, had deteriorated believing the settlement was fair—when it was rigged? How many widows whispered prayers that never rang true?

Then, just as she felt she might collapse into despair, Craig whispered something small—but seismic.

"They've already started revising it. Some players are getting new scores. The court approved changes. They're opening reviews. You may—just may—be able to force them to re-score his case under the new standard."

She swallowed. A tremor of hope stirred in her chest, so delicate she tried to smother it.

They'd covered themselves in legal armor for a decade. They'd assumed silence would always drown the truth. But now, with this information exposed, she saw the fault line in their fortress.

The next move was hers.

And she wouldn't go quietly.

The waiting is its own illness. It fevered the days and chilled the nights, a condition with no blood test and no prescription.

They learned the schedule of bureaucracies the way fans learn schedules for teams—when offices open, when emails tend to arrive, how Fridays are quiet because bad news likes a Monday to spread out in. They learned the topography of hold music. They learned that a denial reads like dust: It settles everywhere and takes a long time to see.

There was a morning she woke to the sound of him calling her by a name that wasn't hers, and for a minute it felt like betrayal.

Then she understood he'd reached into a box of names and pulled the wrong one because the box had no labels left.

She sat on the bed and said her name, softly, the way you remind a child of the street you live on. He blinked.

He asked if the season was over. She said yes. She didn't say which season.

In the afternoons, when the light went weak and wide, he sometimes slipped into a kind of calm that looked like peace if you squinted.

On those days she pulled a shoebox off the closet shelf and took out the programs and credentials he'd saved—laminated badges for tunnels and sidelines and team hotels. She ran her finger down the lists of names and read them to him like prayers. Sometimes his mouth shaped a syllable or two. Sometimes his eyes softened for a beat as if recognizing a place he used to live. Then the softness vanished.

She slid the programs back into their sleeves like dressing a wound.

Bills don't care about memory. They only care about due dates. A man called from the mortgage company and, in a voice that tried to sound compassionate without losing its shape, said words like options and hardship and reinstatement. She wrote them down like vocabulary, then folded the paper and put it under the magnet that used to hold spelling tests. She had a dream that week that the house split down the middle with a long, clean crack and she was the only thing keeping the two halves from sliding into the crawl space. She woke with her arms aching.

The girls invented a game they never told their friends about. They called it "What He Remembers." They'd ask him questions gently—What's Mom's favorite color? What's the dog's name? Where do we keep the forks?—and they'd cheer quietly whenever he found the right answer.

Sometimes he'd ask them for clues, and they'd offer them like gifts: "Starts with B," "rhymes with spoon," "think about the bottom drawer." If the answer didn't come, they changed the subject quickly, as if memory could be spared humiliation.

Craig had explained the way the tests had been scored—how the baseline assumed less in some brains than in others because of the box checked for race, how the past had been baked into the present as if history were destiny and destiny a math problem you couldn't show your work for. He said it'd been embedded in the process, defended by people who didn't have to live with its results, and called objective because that's what you call a blade when you need it to look clean.

She was quiet a long time. Then she said, "So the bar was higher for him."

"Yes. For others like him, too."

She didn't trust her voice enough for another question, so she nodded to herself and let the rage build with the quiet.

News stories began to move differently then. What had once been framed as a triumph of compassion began to fray at the edges.

Reporters said the words out loud. Judges asked other questions. The league released statements that said committed and thorough and ongoing and thanked the court for its leadership. The families released statements that said tired and again and finally.

Somewhere, the math was being redone.

Craig called, voice sounding like someone carrying a fragile box down a flight of stairs.

He told her what he knew, what he could say.

He told her what he couldn't. He told her the court was forcing new standards, that claims would be rescored, that the old math wouldn't be allowed to stand like a stop sign at the end of a bridge that'd already fallen into the river. He asked her to find documents she'd already sent three times and to breathe when she couldn't find them. He said, "We'll try again," and she believed him because for the first time in months someone had said "we" and meant it.

Memory steals nouns first—names, places, the objects that hold a life together. But hope is also a verb. It's the doing of trying again.

She put everything in a clean manila envelope and wrote the address in careful block letters. She asked the clerk to stamp it with the kind of stamp that meant someone had to sign. She wanted a signature on something that week to mean what a signature should.

On nights when the TV was a blue aquarium and his face was the fish moving slowly in it, she'd sit on the floor beside the chair and tell him stories from the middle of their life like lullabies. The night they got lost in a town whose name they still couldn't pronounce. The time he stayed up all night fixing the dishwasher with a YouTube video and a prayer. The Christmas he surprised her with a tree so big they had to cut a hole in the ceiling to stand it upright. He'd look at her sometimes and ask, "Was that us?"

"Yes," she'd say. "It was." And for a moment she'd watch the shape of the man return to his face, the way tide slides sand back into place. Then it'd go again. Tide always goes.

Months later, a check arrived. She paid the mortgage and bought new tires and scheduled the appointment the doctor said couldn't wait another month. She put twenty dollars on a library fine and felt richer, somehow, for the permission to keep borrowing stories that belonged to everyone. She bought a cake from the grocery store bakery with too much frosting and let the girls eat the roses first.

She understood the shape of the bargain in a way she hadn't when she was choking on it: The league had written its protection into their house and then called the arrangement compassionate. The new math changed some numbers. It didn't change the fact that the form had given the pain a signature and told it to be quiet.

Later, after the girls were asleep and the dog had completed his three-circuit patrol of the living room, she stood in the doorway and looked at him. The chair held the body she loved and the mind she missed and somewhere between them was the sound of her own life, steady and astonishing in its persistence. She whispered the three words from the cabinet list—make it through—and then added the word she'd once removed.

Today.

On the news, a panel talked about the future of the game—about safer helmets and protocol improvements and the courage of players who wouldn't be deterred. She turned off the television with the remote taped twice and let the quiet take its place.

Courage could be not quitting on a field. Courage could also be a woman sitting down at a kitchen table with a stack of forms and a pen and a prayer, choosing to live the next sentence. She didn't owe anyone the performance of hope. She owed her girls breakfast in the morning.

Across the country, other kitchens were lit, other chairs occupied by bodies that'd done the work asked of them, other women learning the legal name of what happened to their families. They weren't a movement in the way the news liked movements—no matching signs, no slogans that fit on hats. They were a hum. They were the refrigerator at midnight. They were the baseboard tick when the heat came on. They were what it sounds like when a house keeps being a house after a storm.

She knew tomorrow wouldn't be simple. Simplicity was the kind of word people used when they hadn't read page fourteen of the form. But tomorrow would belong to people who, like her, refused to give the last word to silence.

The league would say the settlement worked. She'd say the settlement taught her how to read a different kind of scoreboard.

One that wasn't measured in yards or dollars, but in the relentless statistics of ordinary grace: mornings risen, meals made, papers filed, breaths taken, glances exchanged that said I'm here, you're here, we're here. Numbers you don't brag about. Numbers you live by.

Somewhere, stadium lights would still come on, fifty-three men would take the field, and a country would rearrange couches and calendars around the spectacle. She didn't begrudge any of it. She knew the seduction of the roar. She also knew what the quiet sounded like when the roar subsided. In this house, the quiet would never be empty again. It'd be the sound of people who learned not to mistake a signature for consent or a check for justice. It'd be the sound of a family refusing to be an asterisk in someone else's press release.

There'd be more forms. There'd be mornings that broke in half by noon. There'd be laughter that surprised them in the produce aisle and tears that came out of nowhere in the dog food aisle, and both would be holy. There'd be one more game on the television with the volume low, and she'd sit on the arm of the chair and ask him who he thought would win, and he'd say the name of a team that wasn't playing, and she'd say, "Good call," and they'd both smile because sometimes truth and kindness had to trade places for a while.

If anyone asked her what justice looked like, she'd tell them it looked like a kitchen table with a pen that didn't skip and a paragraph without a trap door and a phone that got answered by someone who could make a decision. She'd tell them it looked like a scoring system that didn't tie a man's worth to the box checked for race or the neighborhood coded into a ZIP, like a doctor's note that wasn't audited by someone who'd never had to hold a body through a seizure. She'd tell them it looked like more than a check. She'd tell them it looked like her girls getting to be girls.

And if anyone asked her what hope sounded like, she'd tell them it sounded like this house. The hum. The tick. The quiet that wasn't empty anymore. The sentence that wasn't a sentence, but a beginning.

14

MEASURE OF A MAN

PHILADELPHIA: SPRING 2018

What is the measure of a man?

ON December 7, 1943, Freeman White was born. Years later, his biggest dream came true. He'd be drafted by the New York Giants and become a tight end in the National Football League. When he played in the NFL, he didn't know in July 2013 he'd be diagnosed with Alzheimer's disease. Nor that five years later, on a rainy May day in 2018, his time here would end.

Freeman was a man of integrity, honor, faith. Quietly strong, gentle in spirit, selfless in heart. When he walked into a room, you felt steadiness return. The kind of steadiness the world rarely gives back.

When Freeman was diagnosed, the NFL lawsuit was in full gear. Years later, after final approval, I filed a claim for this gentle giant. We waited for the approval letter. It arrived months later, soon after Freeman passed.

Before filing, I noticed we were missing one required form—a third-party verification of his functional decline. Under settlement rules, that statement couldn't be written by family; it had to come from someone who knew the player well enough to attest to his decline. A strange requirement, I thought. But strange was the language of this settlement.

By then Freeman couldn't communicate; Alzheimer's had already begun its cruel work. So his wife, Sally, did most of the talking. I never met her in person, but felt I'd known her forever. She was devoted to Freeman—steady, relentless, loyal. A woman whose faith had hardened into endurance. I could hear it in her voice: fatigue tucked beneath hope.

Sally was strong-willed, skeptical about the process.

"Craig," she told me, "These people don't care about men like Freeman. They'll find a reason to say no."

I reassured her. Freeman had a confirmed Alzheimer's diagnosis from a reputable neurologist in Kansas City. Everything was done by the book.

"Don't worry," I said. "This is exactly what the settlement was built for."

I believed that then. I needed to.

Days later, the third-party statement came from Freeman's lifelong friend William, also from Kansas City. He wrote from the heart:

"Freeman and I have been friends for over 30 years. When I met him, he was a very happy and easy-going man, joyful over the small and large happenings in his life. I would bring my family down to visit him and Sally. We spent many nights sitting and talking politics, social issues, current events and just plain banter.

During this time my wife passed. Freeman provided a valuable resource to me as I raised my two daughters. His knowledge, wisdom and quiet strength provided a comforting source of solace. He is probably more responsible for my daughters' passion for the Kansas City Chiefs than I was.

Today that spark of consciousness is not as bright. This has been a slow progressive process. I have been with Freeman on his good days when he could keep up with a conversation as long as it didn't get too complicated. Other days communication was labored or nonexistent . . . there are times when he did not seem to be cognizant of the fact that he needed to act on a situation.

Is this Alzheimer's endgame? A slow loss of a person's sense of self, their spirit, their soul. He has yet to forget his children's names, or my daughters or thankfully me."

I read that line—"a slow loss of a person's sense of self, their spirit, their soul"—half a dozen times. It stayed with me, sacred. I thought of my grandmother, who'd passed from Alzheimer's years earlier. I remembered the emptiness in her voice, her eyes. Freeman was no different.

Freeman's claim should have been simple.

When the letter arrived in July 2018, my eyes went straight to the bold header: NOTICE OF DENIAL OF MONETARY AWARD CLAIM

I scanned the page for the reason. Section II: "Explanation of Determination." The words were bureaucratic, bloodless, absurd. The Administrator concluded that Freeman's Alzheimer's disease "may have been caused by other factors," including "a potential vitamin B12 deficiency."

That's how the system dismissed a man's life—with a vitamin.

I sat staring at the letter, paper trembling in my hands. After everything this man had given—his body, his mind, his memories—the League reduced him to a deficiency.

I called Sally. She didn't cry at first. Too angry for tears.

"How dare they," she said, her voice shaking. "How dare they tell me he's not sick enough. I've watched him disappear."

I told her we'd fight. And we did. We gathered new medical records, resubmitted reports, sent letters and affidavits. Long nights on the phone with Sally, going over every line of the claim, every test result, every signature. Sometimes she'd pause mid-conversation, whisper:

"He's empty. They stole part of his life—and ours."

It broke me every time.

We filed again. But we couldn't beat Goliath. Freeman's claim was denied again by a system that never intended justice in the first place, no matter what they say in the press.

I've seen denials—legal, professional, personal—but this one cut differently. Because it wasn't just about money. It was about recognition. About dignity. It was the system looking at Freeman and saying, we don't believe you. And to Sally: we don't believe you either.

The injustice wasn't loud. No headlines, no outrage. It came in silence—in the quiet way hope dies when no one's looking.

Sally called me the day the second denial arrived. She didn't sound angry. Just tired.

"It's like they're erasing him, piece by piece," she said. "First his memory, now his worth."

There's a verse: The meek inherit the earth. But it doesn't say when. Sally reminded me of that—her strength wrapped in sorrow. She said faith wasn't about believing everything would be made right—just about believing.

When Freeman passed, I sat at my desk, thought about William's letter again. "A slow loss of self, spirit, and soul." That's what this process had become—for Freeman and hundreds like him.

The league liked to talk about finality, about closure. But closure for whom? Freeman's story was never about finality. It was about a system that decided which lives were valid and which weren't. A system that saw paperwork instead of people.

I still think about Sally—our last conversation, when she thanked me for fighting.

"You did what you could," she said. "That's more than most."

I told her she did too. Love enduring through loss is the purest courage. She said she still prayed every morning—not for justice anymore, but for peace.

"Peace," she said, "for him. For me. For all of them."

And I think of Freeman. His kindness. His humility. The way people spoke his name like a blessing. He was the measure of what a man should be. The league never saw that. They couldn't. Systems don't recognize souls.

The claims process was supposed to bring justice. What it delivered was arithmetic. It measured worth in paperwork, not humanity. Every denial, every excuse, every "vitamin deficiency" was another way of saying: We refuse to see you.

If justice means truth, the truth is this: Freeman was more than a claim. Sally was more than a name on a form. And the men like them—the ones fading quietly in living rooms across the country—were the heart of what this case was supposed to protect.

There's another verse I think of often: The last shall be first, and the forgotten shall be remembered. I like to believe it's true. That somewhere beyond this world of forms and filings, Freeman remembers again. That he's whole. That Sally's prayers didn't vanish into the silence.

Because justice without compassion isn't justice at all. It's procedure dressed as virtue. And I've seen too much of it to mistake one for the other.

Freeman's story was one of many. The names change, but the pattern doesn't. Denials justified by paperwork. Delays disguised as fairness. Families left holding the weight of love with no place to set it down.

In the end, the measure of a man isn't the verdict written in a file. It's the lives he touched. The love he left behind. The way people remember him long after the system stops pretending to care.

That's the truth they can't seal, can't bury, and can't deny.

15

CHAINS

SAN DIEGO, CALIFORNIA: SPRING 2016

Trapped by the system.

THE building looked nice from the outside—freshly painted, shrubs clipped neat, a flag snapping in the wind. But the air inside was different. It smelled of bleach and loneliness. The walls were a soft beige, trying too hard to calm people who'd given up on calm. Faces shuffled past, eyes empty, bodies drifting down hallways that felt like purgatory.

The receptionist smiled mechanically. The fluorescent lights hummed above like a nervous system gone haywire. I followed a nurse past rooms with cracked doors—televisions murmuring, each tuned to a different channel, none watched.

I was there to see a client named Allan. He was fifty-six, a retired player who'd once been a storm on the field—relentless, bruising, unstoppable. The kind of linebacker who could make an entire sideline flinch before the snap. When he hit, you felt it three rows up.

After football, he became a successful financial advisor. He wore tailored suits, quoted market trends, and lectured rookies about planning for the future.

"Don't be the guy who loses it all," he'd tell them. "Play smart when the game's over."

But the game never really ended. It just changed shape.

Now, barely fifty-six, Allan's thoughts were mostly suicidal. His depression was as deep as the hits he once gave. The only things that rivaled it were his memory loss and his frequent episodes of rage. He was trapped in a place meant for the forgotten—a holding pen between life and the slow drift away from it.

The nurse pushed through double doors that hissed, sealing the place.

"Good morning, Mr. C," she said softly, like speaking too loudly might crack someone.

TVs murmured from alcoves. A man argued with a wall. Another stared at a plastic plant as if waiting for it to bloom. Somewhere, a microwave beeped and no one claimed the food.

Allan's hands were still the size of shovels, his knuckles a topography of Sundays. He tried to talk football with the nurse, and for a while he lit up—retelling a story about his first touchdown, the roar of the crowd, the weightless ecstasy of immortality. You could see it land—the memory coming clean for once, the way a spiral sits in your palms and everything makes sense.

Then his voice broke. Tears rolled from his eyes. He drifted back to a day before entering the facility, a moment with his grown son. In anger and confusion, his son—who didn't understand the invisible disease—lashed out, throwing a length of raw chain across Allan's body. It left welts, scars that outlived the bruises.

"He thought I was weak," Allan whispered, tears spilling.

The words hollowed the air. Weakness wasn't his. It belonged to a league that had known the truth and buried it in contracts, profits, and silence.

I looked around at the men lost inside themselves and thought about what kind of chain held a man like Allan here. Not the steel one his son threw, but the invisible one forged by denial—each link binding greed to consequence.

A therapist passed by with a cart of puzzles—thousand-piece skies and oceans with all the blue pieces mixed.

"Keeps the hands busy," she said, and smiled at Allan like busy could stand in for whole.

I sat in silence, watching him pick at the edges of a puzzle piece, his brow furrowed like a man still studying game film. Every few minutes he'd mutter something about practice, about plays, about "getting back out there." His body still remembered the rhythm of preparation, even if his mind had let it go.

Then, as though pulled from another life, I thought about Kevin.

The same disease in a different form.

The next day, my cell phone rang.

ALS had finally taken control and won the battle. Kevin was gone. After a six-year fight, ALS had claimed what football had already stolen.

I sat gripping the phone as though I could crush death itself. My thoughts went to Joyce—his wife—their children, his parents. How do you explain to kids that their father's strength—the thing they trusted more than gravity—is gone?

I remembered the last time I'd seen him. His body was failing, betraying him inch by inch, but his eyes burned with fight. Ironically, one of Kevin's last requests was a scribbled note on a piece of paper to his family that simply said:

Don't let that son of a bitch get a penny.

He was talking about Steve Roberts, his high-profile attorney from Miami who had clawed at the case like a vulture.

Years earlier, Kevin and I sat together and discussed the class action. As much as he wanted me to represent him, he had already signed a retainer agreement that a stranger named Steve Roberts had mailed to him. When Roberts learned Kevin wanted me as his attorney, he went berserk. He either didn't know our friendship or didn't care.

Kevin hated it. He felt uncomfortable. I eased his apprehension, told him to go with Roberts.

"It's all the same," I said.

But Kevin knew better. His note—his last words to his family—weren't about disease or pain. They were about betrayal. They were about Roberts's greed.

And betrayal came quickly.

Kevin fought to the end—not just for his dignity, not just for justice, but for his children's future. He made it clear in his final days that Steve Roberts should never touch a penny. Kevin's dying hand scrawled words carrying the weight of a final will: I don't want Roberts to get anything. The NFL is going to pay him millions from the common benefit fund.

The ink on Kevin's death certificate was barely dry when Roberts moved. As soon as Kevin passed, Roberts presented Kevin's father with a fresh retainer agreement. Inside it was the poison clause—40 percent of his recovery.

Kevin's father, shattered by grief, believed this issue had been resolved. He thought the attorney had honored his son's dying wishes. But he soon discovered Roberts still believed he was entitled to claim millions from Kevin's settlement—the very money Kevin wanted reserved for his children.

The betrayal landed like a blow.

Kevin had fought through ALS, sat in courtrooms, stood before cameras, given his failing body as living testimony to the dangers of the game. He was the face of the concussion litigation. Yet even in death, his legacy wasn't safe. The vultures circled.

When the story broke, it exploded across national media. Headlines screamed: Attorney accused of seeking double payment for representing Kevin Turner in NFL concussion settlement. Kevin's father filed a motion before Judge Anita Brody, accusing Roberts of attempting the unthinkable—double-dipping.

Roberts already had access to the common benefit fund—$112 million set aside to compensate attorneys for their work in securing the settlement. But for Roberts, that wasn't enough. He wanted Kevin's personal award, too, clawing at the $5 million that was meant for Kevin's children. Forty percent of it—millions that would never buy a wheelchair, never cover medical care, never put food on the table.

Kevin begged Roberts in his final months to resolve the dispute. Roberts told him not to worry, that he'd "do the right thing." But when Kevin was gone—when he could no longer speak for himself—Roberts revealed his true intentions. He reached out to Kevin's grieving father asking for a signature, as if paperwork could erase Kevin's dying words.

The national media called Roberts. He gave no comment. They called O'Malley and were told Chris was "unavailable."

The silence was damning.

After bitter legal wrangling, the court reduced Roberts's fee. But he walked away with money Kevin never wanted him to touch—millions from the common benefit fund and a piece of the very award meant for Kevin's children.

The irony cut like a knife. Kevin had given his body to football, his spirit to the cause, his final breath to protecting his children's inheritance. And yet, greed found a way to reach into his grave.

Roberts knew the truth: He was already entitled to millions through the fund. The NFL itself was paying him, just as it was paying O'Malley, Rockman, and the rest of the appointed counsel. Kevin knew it too. That's why his last words were so clear: Don't let him take from me, because he's already taking from them.

But greed is never satisfied. The fund wasn't enough. Roberts wanted both. He wanted the safety net and the spoils. He wanted to be paid twice—once by the League and once by the dying man whose body had been destroyed to make the League rich.

The system allowed it. That was the dirtiest truth of all. Judge Brody presided as gatekeeper, but her rulings consistently favored the architects of the deal. Challenges were smothered, objections brushed aside. So long as the structure of the settlement stood, the insiders—those seated at the table when the $112 million pie was cut—could feast as they pleased.

Kevin's fight became a case study in betrayal. Even in death, he was not safe from the men in suits. His children were not protected from the paper claws of an attorney who had already struck gold. His wishes weren't sacred enough to silence the hunger of men who saw clients not as human beings, but as commodities.

Roberts's betrayal wasn't just about one man. It was a window into the rot at the heart of the entire settlement—the feeding trough that the common benefit fund became. Men like Roberts, O'Malley, and others circled like hyenas, fighting not over justice, but over how much flesh they could tear from the carcass.

And that was the cruelest irony: The very settlement meant to provide justice for men like Kevin had, in practice, provided riches for the lawyers who claimed to stand beside them. Greed had become the quiet engine of the deal. Roberts was just one face of it, but they all drank from the same fountain.

Back in San Diego, Allan believed he had missed team curfew.

"I missed curfew?" he asked the nurse.

She glanced at him with that look—half pity, half apology for the world.

In the next room, the rec-room TV blared Sunday football. The closed captioning called the action like poetry gone wrong: MAN RUNS. MAN FALLS. CROWD CHEERS. A janitor mopped in figure eights while a patient in slippers clapped for touchdowns that were years old. What neither saw were the Post-it notes some announcers were using—retired players turned broadcasters. They too were experiencing depression and memory loss, but you'd never know it from the broadcast.

The next morning, I drove to the Jersey Shore. The Atlantic stretched like an old scar—vast, permanent, silent. The wind salted my face. I thought about chains—how they're built link by link, how they hold ships, how they bind prisoners, how they can pull a man from a ditch or drag him into one. I thought about Allan's son and that length of raw chain, the way grief swings when it doesn't know where to land.

Several days later, I spoke to Kevin's wife, Joyce. I told her he was brave. Not the Hollywood kind. The kind where you wake up inside a failing body and still choose tenderness ten times a day. The kind where you write a note that guards your children even when you know you won't be there to.

I thought about the chains again—metal and metaphorical. The ones we wear willingly because they look like credentials. The ones we're handed because we were too busy helping to ask for a key. The ones we forge ourselves out of silence.

Because silence is the strongest link of all.

Sometimes the only way to break a chain is to put your hands on it and pull.

And sometimes you realize the chains were never yours—they were built by a system that pretended to honor the fallen while cashing their checks. Kevin's note was his rebellion; Allan's tears were his. And mine—mine was this fight.

These weren't isolated tragedies. They were evidence. Every link, every bruise, every betrayed promise was proof of how far the game had strayed from its players.

In the end, we're all chained to something—memory, money, loyalty, loss.

But if you pull hard enough, sometimes, just sometimes, the metal gives way.

16

THE FUND

PHILADELPHIA: SPRING 2018

Greed institutionalized.

WHEN I sat down with Gene Rockman in Philadelphia to discuss a possible NFL action, the conversation turned quickly to money.

Not the players' money.

Not the settlement dollars that might one day trickle down to sick men and grieving families.

No—the conversation was about legal fees.

It wasn't an afterthought or a side note. It was the air in the room.

Rockman laid out the standard structure. Class-action lawyers, he explained, work on contingency. If the players recovered, then we, the lawyers, would take a percentage of that recovery. Simple. Familiar. That was how the business worked.

What he didn't say—and what I'd only later understand—was that beneath that familiar arrangement lived another system. Quieter. Far more lucrative. Far more dangerous.

It was called the common benefit fund.

This fund didn't belong to the players. Not one penny would land in their hands. It was money from the NFL—specifically for the lawyers.

On paper, it was practical: a way to cover the enormous costs of a case this size—experts, travel, depositions, endless drafts of briefs and arguments. In reality, it became something else. Not reimbursement, but fuel. Not support, but motive.

Whoever controlled the fund controlled everything. Who got paid. How much. Whose work mattered and whose didn't.

It was a throne. And only a select few ever saw the steps leading up to it.

To the players, the fund was invisible. They never saw it, never touched it, and most never even heard of it. They were focused on their own claims—on whether the system would recognize their dementia, their memory loss, their blackouts, their ALS. They waited for medical testing, for treatment, for the checks that might keep the lights on or pay for one more round of medication.

But behind the scenes, something else was happening.

While the players lined up for neuropsych exams and baseline testing, a second contest raged over fees. The common benefit allocation became its own separate litigation, with its own alliances, its own betrayals, its own quiet war.

The players had no seat at that table.

They didn't even know the table existed.

That's what made it so dangerous.

After final approval, O'Malley filed a petition with the court asking for $112.5 million in attorney's fees for the handful of lawyers who had, in his words, "secured this historic settlement."

The judge approved the request.

Then she handed O'Malley the keys.

O'Malley—and O'Malley alone—would decide how to divide the $112.5 million. Judge, jury, and executioner.

That was when the truth finally stepped out of the shadows.

It didn't matter how many players I'd sat with, how many miles I'd flown, how many hours I'd spent educating families and securing their endorsement of the deal. In the end, it wasn't about the work.

It was about who held the knife. And O'Malley held it tight.

The distribution process initially looked fair.

Every lawyer seeking a fee had to file a "declaration"—a sworn statement listing every contribution they'd made to the case. Hours, tasks, hearings, briefs, outreach, travel, strategy. On the surface, it looked like accountability.

Beneath it, it was theater.

Each declaration read like a cross between a legal record and a sales pitch. Some lawyers inflated their roles, padded their hours, burnished their stories until they gleamed. They weren't describing what they'd done. They were auditioning. Auditioning for the right to be paid. Auditioning to be seen as indispensable.

I knew my work spoke for itself, but I also knew my status: outsider to the Select Few. So I didn't take chances.

My declaration—with exhibits—was over a hundred pages.

The audience wasn't the players or the families who'd trusted us. It was one judge and one man: Chris O'Malley.

In that world, to be overlooked was to be invisible. And in a system like this, invisibility meant you might as well not exist.

In my declaration, I laid it out plainly.

At O'Malley's request and direction, I had executed a nationwide outreach and education campaign to inform retired players and their families about the settlement's terms and process—and to secure their endorsement before final approval.

I detailed the hours I'd spent, the state lines I'd crossed, the alumni meetings and conferences calls I'd led with hundreds of players at a time. I didn't just rely on my own words. I attached statements from others: high-profile players, union leaders, respected insiders. A letter from the president of the NFL Alumni Association. A letter from the NFL Players Association.

And then there was the letter from Val Butts.

Val is Marion Butts' wife. Marion played running back in the NFL for the San Diego Chargers, New England Patriots, and Houston Oilers between 1989 and 1995. He was my client. Marion was suffering from severe dementia, and Val rarely left his side.

She had spent years fighting the NFL on everything—disability, workers' compensation, basic recognition of what the game had done to her husband. She had testified in ways the public never saw, advocated behind the scenes, turned her life into a battlefield for fairness.

Her letter to Judge Brody was long, raw, and precise. Marion had seen a neurologist at thirty-one and was diagnosed with permanent neurological damage and dementia. She described Social Security declaring him permanently disabled in 2002. She described the isolation of families who were fighting alone, ashamed to admit what was happening inside their homes.

And then she described the call she made to me at 9:38 a.m. on September 13, 2013—how that call "changed the course of our lives."

She told the judge I was the only lawyer who had spent years traveling the country to educate players and their families—who took the time to explain the settlement in plain language, to help them decide whether to stay in or opt out. She wrote that without my efforts, thousands of players might have walked away from the deal altogether, terrified of signing away rights they didn't fully understand.

She wrote about something even more important than money: that I treated every player the same, whether I represented him individually or not. That I was their advocate, not just their lawyer. That my vigilance and knowledge had given them something they rarely felt: solace.

Val's words weren't just testimony. They were a plea on behalf of every family that had been waiting years for someone—anyone—to stand next to them instead of in front of them.

In a fair system, a letter like that would have mattered.

But in the world of the fund, the voices of players and families became footnotes. What mattered was power—who controlled it, who O'Malley chose to elevate, and who he decided to erase.

O'Malley's $112.5 million petition stripped away any pretense of fairness. It wasn't just about compensating work—it was about consolidating influence.

He used the fund as a weapon and a reward. It elevated him, rewarded allies, and punished dissent. It institutionalized greed.

For me, it became brutally personal.

I had spent years walking into players' homes—listening to wives describe the men they had lost, watching children study their fathers like strangers. I carried those stories into courtrooms and meeting rooms. I did the work most of the Select Few wouldn't touch. I traveled, explained, reassured, answered the same questions a hundred times so players could sign on—or walk away—with eyes open.

Those efforts helped secure the 99.1 percent endorsement the court leaned on so heavily to approve the deal. Without their buy-in, there would have been no settlement.

I thought that meant something.

But when the fund was divided, justice wasn't in the room.

Power was. Ego. Appetite.

O'Malley gave himself close to $65 million. He set aside more for his own future. Then he carved up the rest like spoils of war, feeding his long-term allies while leaving others to starve.

I was one of the ones left to starve.

I wasn't cut out entirely—that might have been easier. Instead, I was handed a nominal amount—less than $1 million. Not enough to cover the litigation-funding debt I'd taken on in reliance upon his promises. Not enough to come close to the contribution he'd privately assured me would be mine.

It was a bone tossed after the feast.

It stung. Not just because of the money—though years of work were dismissed in a spreadsheet cell—but because of what it revealed.

I had believed, maybe foolishly, that this fight was about justice. That if I sat in enough kitchens and union halls, if I heard enough stories and carried them faithfully, the system would care. That the truth would matter.

But in the end, it didn't.

The players' pain justified the fund's size. Their stories were paraded when convenient, then shelved. The men whose bodies had paid the price became invisible again the moment the checks for lawyers started printing.

Meanwhile, the players kept waiting. The online portal spun. Denials and audits piled up like snowdrifts. The same men whose names had been invoked to justify the fund now fought for basic recognition—arguing over definitions, timelines, and "objective measures" that shifted like smoke.

That contrast is the part I can't shake.

In one room, a single stroke of a pen could move $65 million.

In another, a wife needed three separate notarized letters to prove her husband had forgotten where the forks were kept.

Kevin Turner's story was another lesson. Even in death, his last wish—that Steve Roberts never touch a dime of his recovery—was betrayed. Roberts, already positioned to receive millions from the common benefit fund, still tried to take 40 percent of Kevin's personal award.

It was greed in its purest form, mirroring the system that allowed the fund to exist.

The common benefit fund had become a shadow economy. A second settlement stacked behind the first—this one for the lawyers.

People sometimes ask if I regret it. The meetings, the miles, the late-night calls, the belief that truth would count for something.

I don't regret the work.

I regret the lesson.

I regret learning that in a system like this, truth is a currency you can spend, but not redeem.

Still, there's always a turning point—anger cooling into something sharper. I stopped asking whether the fund was fair. I started documenting what it revealed.

I saved the emails. Kept the letters. Wrote down dates, names, and who told me never to put anything in writing. I remembered the tone in their voices and the way rooms felt when conflict of interest was being dressed up as procedure.

Because one day, the story of the fund would not be told in the language of sealed orders and redacted lines. It would be told in the language of people. Of players. Of families.

And that story would need a witness.

In the end, I walked away from the allocation with two truths braided tight:

The players were still waiting.

And so was I.

Not waiting for the system to deliver. That illusion was gone.

I was waiting for the moment when the truth could no longer be buried in footnotes and sealed filings. When someone would pull back the curtain on how greed had been institutionalized in the very case that promised justice.

Someone had to tell that story.

And I knew, deep down, that someone was me.

17

THE THRILL OF VICTORY AND THE AGONY OF DEFEAT

COMMUNITIES AROUND THE COUNTRY: PRESENT DAY

Time.

IT turned out the real opponent was never the NFL, or the lawyers, or even the diseases themselves. It was time—silent, relentless, undefeated. It stripped players of memory and language, of the parts of themselves that once filled every room they walked into.

Time ticked in waiting rooms where the magazines were three years old. It ticked in kitchens where pillboxes sat on the counter like tiny calendars of surrender. It ticked between questions at neuropsych exams—What day is it? Who is the president? Can you count backward by sevens?—and in the long pauses wives learned to leave so their husbands could search a little longer for answers that once lived on the tip of their tongues. It lived in the hallway at 3 a.m., when a man stood barefoot in the dark and couldn't remember which door led to his own bedroom.

By mid–2025, the stories were everywhere if you knew how to look. Former stars stumbled through grocery-store aisles, forgetting what they came for. Fierce linebackers couldn't button their shirts. Quarterbacks once praised for field vision now stared at walls, lost in fog. Many of their claims had been denied.

In Ohio, a wife taped notes around the house—Milk in fridge above the handle, Your keys are in the bowl by the front door—until the walls looked like a scavenger hunt for a life that used to be obvious. In Florida, a daughter installed locks higher on the doors after her father wandered outside at midnight and rang the bell like a guest. In Texas, a son set his alarm for 5 a.m. so he could hide the family shotgun before school. For every story, the League had an answer: Wrong form, not from head trauma. Exaggeration.

And yet, on Sundays, the machine churns on.

Fans roar, anthems play, networks roll out highlight packages of fresh heroes being minted in real time. Stadiums shake with joy. Touchdowns exploded in fireworks and choreographed end-zone dances. The agony of yesterday was erased by the thrill of today.

Drone shots swooped over full parking lots. Graphics flashed. America exhaled. Monday-morning shows debated legacies and playoff pictures. Nobody ran highlight reels of wives counting pills or kids learning how to pronounce frontotemporal degeneration for a school counselor. The soundtrack of the sport drowned out the metronome of decline.

But beneath the noise, the cost was everywhere, it still is.

On September 29, 2022, I remember watching as the Miami Dolphins sent quarterback Tua Tagovailoa back onto the field just four days after a concussion. Millions saw what happened next: His fingers seized and curled grotesquely as he lay on the turf (known as a "fencing response"), his nervous system broadcasting what the League had spent years trying to bury. It was one of the most chilling images football had ever produced. (Tagovailoa would miss the next two weeks, though would suffer another concussion on December 25, ruling him out for the rest of the season.)

Still, nothing meaningful changed.

Thousands of retired players lived with migraines, tremors, rage, and depression, yet were systematically excluded from recovery—financially, medically, spiritually. The NFL had mastered plausible deniability, the art of legal maneuvering, the practice of burying pain beneath paperwork.

I sat with men who had played through darkness because the culture insisted pain was the toll. They told me about smelling salts and dark rooms, about coaches calling it "getting your bell rung," trainers holding up two fingers and asking how many because one finger was too easy. Now those same men submitted to portals and protocols, to audits and appeals—a new kind of gauntlet where the hits were paperwork and the bruises didn't show.

And still, they remained America's heroes.

That was the paradox: The very men being discarded were the same ones still celebrated in NFL Films montages and anniversary specials. They had given their blood, their minds, their futures to the game, and in return they received silence, delay, and dismissal.

Chris O'Malley received something else.

As lead counsel and self-appointed treasurer of the common benefit fund, he authorized more than $65 million to his own firm—courtesy of the NFL. The lawyer who presented himself as the players' fiercest advocate became the League's greatest asset. He got what he wanted.

The players got promises. Paper. Time.

And me?

I had to face a truth more painful than any order a judge could sign or any headline the media could print: I had sold the deal.

I had flown from city to city, stood in front of broken men and their families, and told them this settlement was their salvation. I believed it—until I couldn't.

Empty promises.

Empty words.

Empty pockets.

There was a night in a Newark hotel when that truth finally stopped knocking and kicked in the door.

My suitcase lay open on the bed, zipper teeth grinning like a wound. Next to it sat an itinerary that used to feel like mission and now felt like indictment—Houston. Phoenix. Minneapolis. Canton. I could still see the faces: a center whose hands shook as he signed his name, a cornerback who couldn't remember the route to his own front porch, a wide receiver who apologized to his eight-year-old son for forgetting his birthday, then apologized again for forgetting that he had forgotten.

I wondered what my speeches sounded like in their kitchens now—comfort, or betrayal?

I'd gotten involved in the litigation because I thought I was helping. I thought I was delivering justice. But in the end, without realizing it, I had been delivering silence wrapped in promises that could never be kept.

I had become part of the machine.

The machine isn't gears and cogs. It's incentives. It's who gets invited into meetings and who hears about decisions after the fact. It's who's told, "Never put that in writing," and who holds the ledger anyway. It's the soft tyranny of "That's just how it works" and the hard fact of who gets paid. It's the way a number like 99.1 percent can be both miracle and muzzle.

Looking back, I see it clearly: The NFL never truly feared the lawsuit. They feared the truth. They feared players telling their stories in open court, on witness stands, under oath. They feared the raw humanity that statistics and contracts could never sanitize.

So they settled. They paid. They bought silence.

Settlement is an interesting word. It sounds like peace. It sounds like a small town where people plant gardens, hang wind chimes, and wave from porches. But for the men I met, settlement meant survival on a stopwatch. It meant proving your own deterioration according to someone else's rubric. It meant releasing the League from the very harm that left you needing help—while your signature still shook from the effort of remembering how to hold a pen.

And I helped them sign.

There's a photo on my phone I can't bring myself to delete. A banquet hall in a Midwestern city. Folding chairs in rows. A projection screen at the front with a slide titled What This Means for You. In the second row, a man sits with his hands folded, wedding ring glinting under fluorescent light. His wife sits beside him, chin lifted, eyes rimmed red. I remember their names. They endorsed the settlement because I asked them to. They thanked me afterward.

When I called months later to check on them, the number had been disconnected.

I didn't understand it then. But intent doesn't erase impact. Good men can be used.

And I was used.

The strangest quiet in my life came when the fight ended. It wasn't the peace I imagined, but a hollow silence that felt like punishment.

For seven years, concussions consumed me. This wasn't just a case; it was a crusade. I woke up thinking about it, fell asleep with filings open on my desk, and traveled so much that hotel rooms began to feel more familiar than home. I worked through holidays and birthdays, through nights when my kids asked why I couldn't stay for dinner. Every mile, every late-night call, every hearing felt like another brick in a wall I didn't realize I was building between myself and the rest of my life.

I believed the system would eventually recognize what we were doing—that truth and courage, fought for hard enough, could still move a court. I wasn't part of a mega-firm with endless reserves; I was a man with conviction and a belief that doing the right thing still mattered.

To stay in the ring, I borrowed money from a litigation funder—money I was told carried "no real risk." Use it for travel, for outreach, for players' meetings, they said. Pay it back when the fees come in. It sounded safe.

Risk is like rot. It hides behind the wallpaper until the whole structure collapses.

When the common benefit fund was finally carved up, I waited for fairness. What arrived instead was a lesson. My share was nominal—so small it couldn't even pay off the principal, let alone the interest, on the debt I'd taken to keep fighting. I remember staring at the numbers, not in shock but instead with recognition. I had seen this play before—this exact hit—only now I was the one lying on the field.

The very fund that was supposed to honor sacrifice became the arena for a quiet betrayal. The man who had orchestrated it—the same one who talked about brotherhood and "common benefit"—carved the fund like a carcass, leaving scraps for the lawyers who had done the hard work in the trenches.

For seven years, I practiced nothing else. My firm withered. Old clients moved on. The phones that once rang with opportunity now collected on debt. I sold what I could, cut what I couldn't, and kept telling myself that someday it would make sense, that I'd look back and call it worth it.

But when the big checks cleared for others and the doors closed on me, I realized "justice" had been repackaged as a product.

The fallout came slowly, like erosion.

I lost my savings—including the money I'd put aside for my children's education, and the retirement fund that had once been my quiet reassurance. Each dollar I'd saved became another casualty of my faith in the system. I lost time—our only nonrenewable asset. My family carried more than they should have had to bear.

There were nights when I pulled into my driveway after court and stayed in the car, unable to walk inside. I wasn't ashamed because I'd done something wrong; I was ashamed because I'd done everything right and still lost.

People ask what it was all for. What cause, what principle, what promise justified giving everything I had?

The answer, as much as it hurts, is simple: I believed.

I believed integrity could still win inside a courtroom and out. I believed loyalty and decency would be honored. I believed that if I fought hard enough, the truth would find daylight. That belief cost me nearly everything—my practice, my financial security, and nearly my family.

Thank God love is sometimes stronger than reason. My wife stood beside me through all of it, even when there was nothing left to stand on.

The irony is that I wasn't naïve. I'd seen greed up close for years. I'd watched men use the law as leverage and justice as the-ater. But I never imagined that the people preaching "juatice" would weaponize the phrase. The fund was supposed to represent fairness—a recognition of shared sacrifice. Instead, it became a monument to hypocrisy.

I was left buried beneath the same machinery I had once helped build.

My downfall wasn't bad strategy. It was trust. Trusting O'Malley. Trusting Rockman. Trusting that the men leading the charge still cared about the players, about the purpose. Trusting that "common good" was more than a line in a brief.

That trust was my undoing.

But even as the walls fell, one pillar remained: The truth wouldn't stay buried.

I didn't know if anyone would care or listen, but I knew I would tell it. Silence—no matter how understandable—would make me complicit. I had watched too many men lose everything while the people who claimed to speak for them profited from their pain.

Maybe I lost most of what the world calls success, but I didn't lose my conviction. The players had given their bodies. I had given my time, and I still believe what I often tell others:

Time is our biggest asset. When someone else takes it from you, it can never be replaced.

In the end, we were all part of the same story—a story about what happens when loyalty meets greed and truth is traded for power. I didn't set out to be part of the evidence, but that's what I became.

Justice never truly came for the players. Not real justice. The league raised its glasses. O'Malley cashed his $65 million check. Across America, wives hid guns, children whispered in fear, and men stared into mirrors and didn't recognize the faces looking back.

The thrill of victory had vanished long ago. All that remained was the agony of defeat.

And justice—true justice—vanished with it.

Defeat, though, has its own chemistry. It strips away vanity, dissolves excuse, and leaves only what refuses to go quietly.

Somewhere between the denials and the declarations, between the envelopes marked FINAL and the phone calls that began with "I'm sorry," another certainty took root: The story wasn't over just because the money had moved.

The scoreboard might be turned off, but the game isn't finished.

Time, the undefeated opponent, keeps marching. But time can also be a witness. It preserves what people think they've buried—the emails, the calls, the instructions to keep it off paper, the allocations dressed up as justice. It remembers the wives who wondered which personality of their husband would show up each day, the daughters who sold laptops to pay appeal fees, the players who trusted the wrong people because hope was the only currency they had left.

The league will keep the lights bright on Sundays. The cameras will keep finding joy. That's what the machine does.

But somewhere off camera, the truth is keeping its own ledger. And when the moment comes to read it aloud, I intend to be there—pages in hand, names intact.

Because the real thrill now isn't a touchdown.

It's a reckoning.

And the agony that matters isn't a mark in a loss column. It's what happens when a system asks a man to sign away the right to name what broke him—and silences the other who is fighting to defend that voice.

I can't give the players back their time. No one can. But I can refuse to waste any more of mine pretending that a settlement was a cure.

So I'm done pretending.

The next chapter won't begin in a ballroom or a press conference. It will begin where truth always does:

At a desk.

With a pen.

On the record.

EPILOGUE: AFTER THE NOISE

BACK HOME: FALL 2025

Echoes and warnings.

I STILL have file cabinets full of files marked *asymptomatic* and *diagnosed.* I have the legal briefs I filed over the past several years for the players who could afford the $1,000 appeal payment, and I have the files marked *closed.*

I mostly work remotely now, as I have since COVID. My phone still rings, just not as often, and the calls are usually from an old criminal client or a friend who was stopped and issued a traffic summons. I no longer practice law, I don't believe in justice.

The last few years have been brutal financially. I paid back the litigation funder most of what I borrowed to subsidize my end of the case, but I am still over $1 million in debt. The NFL case has taken my breath away in more ways than one. Relationships with some of my clients have changed; they've grown more reserved, more distant. Many confuse my nominal payment from the common benefit fund with O'Malley's $65 million, assuming a substantial portion of that money ended up in my pocket. With so many of their claims denied, I can understand why they feel that way.

My father used to tell me that things always have a way of working out. He passed unexpectedly in the middle of the NFL litigation, and that's when I learned the second half of that truth: Yes, things always work out—they just may not work out the way you hoped.

My client with the three daughters is now a widow. Her husband passed several years ago. Her youngest daughter is tall enough to reach the top shelf without a stepstool and is breathtakingly beautiful. The oldest has learned how to laugh again without checking the room first. The middle one has a driver's license and a habit of putting the keys in the wrong place and then remembering exactly where she left them—an act of reclamation that feels small and huge at once.

I've seen that even in families where players have finally recovered financially, the hard things haven't stopped. What's changed is that the family has learned how to carry them differently. There are still lists in the drawer and sticky notes on the fridge, routines in ink and rituals in pencil. The television in the corner still lives at a low volume. On Sundays, the sound of the game hovers like a ghost at the edge of the room and then recedes, and nobody pretends that isn't complicated. The chair in the living room still faces the screen at an angle, because the body in the chair remembers how to look at a field even when the mind wanders off without permission.

There are grocery lists that include birthday candles and cake mix. There is a calendar with the words *college visit* and *car inspection* and *call Aunt Nina* and *game night* written in confident marker. There is more future on the wall than there used to be, but in many homes, that future is still uncertain.

What changed outside the players' homes was more than what changed inside. The public now takes concussions seriously—not just in the States, but around the world. At the same time, football remains in the blood of those whose lives have always revolved around it. Some of my friends who are former players have sons who are now on active NFL rosters or fighting to get there.

Sometimes I ask, "Does it bother you that your son plays ball in the league?"

They hesitate, look at me, then shrug it off. "It's just in our blood," they say.

Some things have changed, though.

In 2021, the thing so many families felt but could not name was finally called out in public: race-norming—the idea that a Black man's mind began from a lower baseline; the calculus that assumed less so it could demand more.

That winter, the men in suits did what they do when the sunlight gets too bright: They formed a committee. By March 2022, the court made those committees' promises official. The judge ordered the old math stripped out. Claims would be rescored. Those who had been denied could be re-tested. The door that should never have been locked was, at last, unlocked.

The calls started. Not all at once, not from everyone. But they started. A handful of families heard the word *approved* where once they had heard *insufficient*. Others heard silence, followed by more forms.

On the claim administrator's website and in press releases and interviews, phrases appeared like *course correction*, *eliminating bias*, *ending race-based assumptions*. There were photographs of handshakes. There were numbers that looked impressive until you set them next to the actual lives they were meant to measure.

By 2024, the public tally crossed a round number—more than $1 billion paid out across the country, the kind of statistic that looks clean in headlines and impossible in kitchens. Reporters dug under the figure and found what families already knew: Behind every dollar were rules that bent into denials; the network of approved doctors was thinner than promised; the audit was a machine that sometimes ate the paperwork and then swore it had never seen it.

They put those findings on the front page. The league put out responses that used the word *committed* like a prayer bead. People argued on television. Families sat at tables and waited for the mail.

In 2025, another kind of statement appeared—this one from a national brain injury group that had watched too many cases stall out at the same corner. They said, plainly:

If the doctor in your own network says this man has the illness you promised to pay for, then pay for it. Don't sandbag it with a different doctor's doubt. Don't pretend the process is the point. Make the families whole. Do what you say you will do.

It felt like common sense written in bold, which is to say it felt radical.

None of it undid the damage. Undoing was never on offer. But something else had taken root: the right to name what happened, the right to demand a different arithmetic, the right to insist that the new math not be written with invisible ink. That is not justice, not exactly. But it is at least a path. Paths are how people get somewhere when the bridges are out.

Here is what the present looks like from inside the house:

The man in the chair has good days and bad days. On good days, he is gentle and a little silly. He remembers the old dog's first name and calls the new dog by it on purpose, then laughs because humor is the only way to honor the old dog properly. He asks for pancakes and then forgets to eat them and still compliments them anyway, which is its own kind of grace.

On bad days, he drifts. He asks where his helmet is. He asks if they won. Sometimes he asks where his mother went, and the answer lands like a second funeral.

In other homes, the kitchen table is scarred. The wood has a groove where a nervous hand traced the same loop through years of phone calls. There are flecks of blue ink along the edge where a pen exploded while someone waited for answers. The table holds all of it: denial letters and birthday candles, freedom-of-information drafts and pizza boxes, a stack of essays and another of bills. It is an altar. It is a workbench. It is the place where a family remembers they are a family, not a case number.

In one home, on a shelf next to the photo of him in uniform and the photo of him in a suit and tie and the photo of him in a T-shirt holding a newborn with his whole body bent into a question mark of tenderness, there is a printed copy of the court order that ended race-based baselines. It doesn't look like much—just paper, words in a font that means *serious*. But it represents a door opened and a hallway of rooms that finally let in the light.

Yes, there were headlines about money. Yes, the number passed a billion. Yes, someone on television said the word *success* without flinching. Yes, there were handshakes. Yes, there were lawyers praised and lawyers paid. Yes, there were victories.

And still, the work remains.

Because the truth is that the settlement didn't end anything. It reorganized things. It moved the fight from the field to the form, from Sunday to Monday, from the roar of the stadium to the hush of the waiting room. It gave families a new encyclopedia to learn and then argued with them about pronunciation.

It created new words that do not sound like sickness and somehow are: BAP, Baseline, Appeals, Audit. It built a maze and put signs in it and told people the maze itself was compassion. The people who have to walk it know otherwise. Compassion is not a labyrinth. Compassion is a door propped open and someone saying, "This way. I'll stay with you."

Still, something real did shift. After sunlight found its way into the room where the old math had been done—after people said the quiet part out loud and refused to take it back, after a judge signed and an administrator admitted and even the League used words like *eliminate* and *fix*—Black families saw something they had always deserved: a standard that did not assign them a lower starting line in the name of science.

Files were reopened. Tests were rescored. Some men who had been told, by letter, that their failure to qualify was their own fault were told by a different letter that they qualified after all. I'm sure that the first time a family heard *approved* under the new standard, they cried and then laughed and then cried again.

The approval didn't erase the years. It didn't pay back the interest charged to their hearts. But it said, if only for a moment, that the world had tilted slightly toward fair.

The settlement's machinery still grinds. The plan administrator still issues status reports with charts and graphs and language that shows its work. The doctors still have waiting rooms with televisions bolted high in the corner and stacks of last month's magazines. Appeals still take too long. Audits still feel, at times, like fishing expeditions. Families still plan dinner around phone calls that may or may not come.

But more of those calls end in "Yes." More of those emails carry a number instead of a footnote. More of those footnotes are politely ignored when the number is finally what it should have been in the first place.

Ask around in 2025 and the story is not simple. Some men are the same. Some are worse. Some were never properly diagnosed and happen to be fine. Some were misdiagnosed and paid anyway. Some died without seeing a dollar. Some died with the letter still unopened on the counter.

Most live in the middle.

The middle is not a headline. The middle is where children go to school and someone pays the light bill and someone keeps track of appointments and someone looks at the man in the chair and says, "We're okay," and then walks into the kitchen and cries for exactly fourteen seconds so nobody has to carry it alone.

If there is a lesson in all of this, it's less poetic than people might want. It's this: Systems do not fix themselves. They can be forced into repairs, shamed into upgrades, compelled by courts to stop doing what they should never have done. Left alone, they calcify. They settle into their most comfortable posture—the posture of those who do not have to live with the consequences.

So the families will not leave them alone. Not because they like fighting. Because they like living. Because they remember what life was like before their house became a case study, and they want more of *that* and less of *this* for the people who come after them.

For those who ask what to do now, the answers are practical and unglamorous:

To the League—if a doctor in your own network signs his name, honor it unless you can truly prove something is wrong.

Stop asking for forms you already have. Build the network of physicians in the cities where the players actually live. Publish the numbers without pruning them for optics. Fund the clinics that are already doing the work. Fund the home-health aides who make it possible for the men to stay in the rooms where they built their lives. Fund the people who keep the household ledgers from collapsing. Stop using *fraud* by players as an all-purpose excuse not to pay.

Sometimes the moral arc bends very slowly, and sometimes it bends because someone keeps stepping on it with their whole weight. The bending isn't beautiful. It's bruised. It squeaks.

If you want beauty, look at the way the youngest granddaughter sits on the arm of the chair and tells her grandfather about her day, even when he interrupts to ask which jersey he should wear for a game that ended twenty years ago. If you want redemption, look at the way the child answers the question as if it were the most ordinary thing in the world to be both a kid and a historian at the same time.

There are still journalists circling the story like drones over a floodplain, trying to capture its scope. There are producers who will find ways to put the quiet on a screen—the refrigerator hum, the baseboard tick, the sound a pen makes when it crosses a line that should never have been written. If they are honest, they'll show how the hero does not always look like a man with broad shoulders. Sometimes the hero looks like a woman on hold, a child who knows where the fork drawer is, a neighbor who shows up with a rake and a question about which trash bags the township prefers, because sometimes the miracle is just that the trash gets picked up on time.

This is how *my* story ends, but it is not how *the* story ends. The story will keep going through hearings and orders and revised matrices and updated portals and the slow work of people who refuse to be reduced to footnotes.

It will keep going through college applications and first apartments and weddings and babies who will know their grandfather by the way people say his name. It will keep going through fundraisers and funerals and the kind of living that resists summary. It will keep going because that's what families do: They keep going.

On the shelf, alongside the court order and the photographs, there is one more document now—a letter to the future. It isn't long. It says:

We lived through this. We told the truth about it. If it happens again, may you find us in these pages and in these rooms, not as ghosts but as witnesses. The field was never just a field. The game was never just a game. We are the people who stayed when the lights went out. We are the people who kept the lights on anyway.

The present day is never just an update. It is a promise to the past and a down payment on the future. It is a family in a house that learned the language of forms and refused to let the forms write their story alone. It is a woman who keeps showing up in rooms where decisions are made and says the words that need saying. It is a man who is still here. It is three girls who grew up and did not forget how to play.

It is the quiet, transformed from a sentence into a sanctuary.

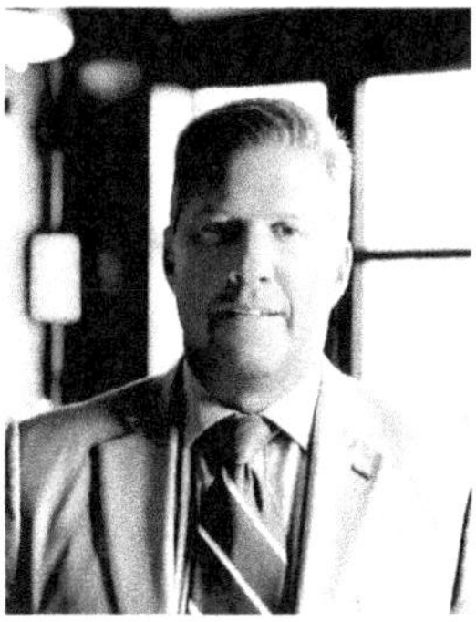

ABOUT THE AUTHOR

Craig Mitnick is a lawyer, entrepreneur, and writer whose career has spanned high-stakes litigation, creative business ventures, and advocacy for those whose voices are too often unheard. Best known for his work representing thousands of retired NFL players in the landmark concussion litigation, Mitnick has built a reputation as a relentless advocate for justice and accountability.

Mitnick received his BBA from Emory University in Atlanta, Georgia, and his law degree from George Washington University in Washington, DC.

Beyond the courtroom, he has founded multiple ventures that merge law, technology, and consumer protection, including innovative platforms designed to give individuals direct access to their rights. His work reflects a lifelong commitment to leveling the playing field—whether in the justice system, in business, or in everyday life.

Mitnick's writing draws deeply on his professional experiences and personal relationships, weaving stories that illuminate both the struggles and the resilience of those caught at the intersection of power, profit, and human cost. His voice—equal parts candid, passionate, and unflinching—offers readers an inside look at the realities of law, sports, and the pursuit of justice in America.

For more about Craig's role in the NFL Retired Players' Concussion Litigation, please see his declaration that was filed in the Federal court for the Eastern District of Pennsylvania.

www.ingramcontent.com/pod-product-compliance
Lightning Source LLC
LaVergne TN
LVHW020414220926
848484LV00018B/2570/J